# Keto Diet

*The Complete Cookbook for Beginners. Lose Weight Healthily with 100 Easy Recipes and a 7-Day Meal Plan.*

Mia Lucas

# TABLE OF CONTENTS


**Introduction** — 1

**Chapter 1: Overview of the Keto Diet** — 5

**Chapter 2: The Benefits of the Keto Diet** — 12

**Chapter 3: Getting Started with the Keto Diet** — 20

**Chapter 4: Breakfast & Brunch Recipe Ideas** — 25

Asiago Bagels — 25

Bacon & Avocado Omelet — 27

Bacon - Egg & Cheese Cups — 29

Bacon & Cheese Frittata — 31

Bacon & Egg Muffins — 33

Bagels & Cheese — 35

Banana Pancakes — 37

Biscuits & Gravy — 39

BLT Wrap — 41

Blueberry Scones — 42

Breakfast Burrito — 44

Brunch Zucchini Bread - Slow-Cooked — 45

Butter Coffee — 47

Cheesy Mushroom Omelet — 48

Choco-Breakfast Waffles 50

Coconut-Almond Egg Wraps 52

Coffee Cake 54

Cream Cheese Eggs 56

Healthy Bacon Hash & Eggs 57

Italian Cheesy Omelet 59

Mackerel & Eggs 61

1-Minute Keto Muffins 63

Sesame - Poppy Seed Bagels 65

**Chapter 5: Lunchtime Favorites** **67**

Avocado - Tuna Melt Bites 67

Baked Zucchini Noodles with Feta 69

Ham & Spinach Mini Quiche 71

Tuna Salad & Chives 73

Tuna Stuffed Avocado 74

Avocado - Corn Salad 75

Caprese Salad 77

Cobb Salad 79

Deviled Chicken Salad Eggs 81

Kale Parmesan Salad 83

Keto Salad Niçoise    84

Lobster Salad    86

Steak Salad    87

Thai Pork Salad    89

Vegetarian Club Salad    91

Asiago Tomato Soup    93

Beef & Carrot Soup - Instant Pot    95

Beef Stew    97

Chicken Chowder - Crockpot    99

Creamy Asparagus Soup    101

Egg Drop Soup    103

Kale - Sausage & Mushroom Soup    105

Mexican Chicken Soup - Slow-Cooked    107

No-Beans Chili Delight    109

**Chapter 6: Poultry Options**    **111**

Asparagus - Stuffed Chicken    111

Basil Stuffed Chicken Breasts    113

Cheesy Chicken Nuggets    115

Chicken Mozzarella & Pesto Casserole    117

Crack Chicken - Slow-Cooked    119

Creamy Onion Chicken                                     121

Preparation Technique:                                   121

Green Beans & Chicken                                    123

Kung Pao Chicken                                         125

Lemon Chicken with Angel Hair Pasta                      127

Oven-Baked Pan-Fried Chicken                             129

Pizza Chicken Casserole                                  131

Rosemary Ranch Chicken Kabobs                            133

Stuffed Chicken with Bacon & Asparagus                   135

**Chapter 7: Beef Options**                              **137**

Bacon Burger Cabbage Stir Fry                            137

Barbacoa Beef – Instant Pot                              139

Beef Pizza                                               141

Cabbage Skillet Tacos                                    143

Cheesy Steak Pinwheels                                   145

Enchilada Skillet Dinner                                 146

Feta-Stuffed Burgers                                     148

Ground Beef Keto Meatballs                               150

Meatloaf                                                 151

Monterey Mug Melt                                        153

Skillet Steak - Nacho Style    154

Slow-Cooked London Broil    156

Spinach-Mozzarella Stuffed Burgers    158

Stroganoff    160

**Chapter 8: Pork & Lamb Options    162**

Bacon & Brussels Sprouts    162

Jamaican Jerk Pork Roast    164

Kalua Pork & Cabbage    166

Pork Kabobs    168

Stuffed Pork Chops    170

Quick & Easy Lamb Chops    172

**Chapter 9: Healthy Dessert Options    174**

Almond Coconut Bars - Instant Pot    174

Almond Pumpkin Seed Bars    176

Amaretti Cookies    178

Blueberry Cupcakes    180

Chocolate Mini Cakes - Instant Pot    182

Chocolate Mousse    184

Easy Brownie Inug    186

No-Bake Coconut Cashew Protein Bars    187

Peanut Butter Protein Bars   189

Pumpkin Bread   191

Pumpkin Cheesecake with Almond Pecan Crust   193

Raspberry Coke – Slow Cooker   195

Raspberry Fudge   197

Strawberry & Cream Cakes   199

Smoothies   201

Almond Lover Smoothie   201

Blueberry - Banana Bread Smoothie   203

Blueberry Essence   205

Cinnamon Smoothie   206

Smoothie in A Bowl   208

Strawberry Avocado with Almond Milk   210

**Chapter 9: 7-Day Meal Plan**   **211**

**Conclusion**   **216**

**Recipes Index**   **221**

**Description**   **227**

# Introduction

Congratulations on purchasing the *Keto Diet: The Complete Cookbook for Beginners. Lose Weight Healthily With 100 Easy Recipes and a 7-Day Meal Plan.* Thank you for doing so.

I have filled it with tons of recipes to suit your desires for breakfast, lunch, dinner, and desserts. Everyone will surely find a new favorite!

Your new 7-day meal plan will provide you with many new ways to change your lifestyle. You will never be hungry and will remain within the constraints of the keto plan.

### How to Begin:

*Step 1:* Choose a non-stressful week to begin the ketogenic diet plan.

*Step 2:* Purge the pantry and fridge.

*Step 3:* Restock the fridge and pantry with ketogenic food items.

*Step 4:* Consider skipping one meal each day. Maybe sleep a little longer and have brunch.

*Step 5:* Initially, don't exceed your net carbs and don't limit the fat and protein you consume.

*Step 6:* Make a routine. Drink a large glass of water and have a supplement of a ½ teaspoon of MCT oil or two teaspoons of coconut oil to get your day started.

*Step 7*: Keep track of your ketone levels.

In many cases, you are currently burning glucose as your 'fuel' source, which in turn will change your food into energy. The remainder of the glucose develops into fat and is stored in your body to be consumed at a later time. The keto diet will set up your body to deplete the stored glucose. Once that is accomplished, your body will focus on diminishing the stored fat you have saved as fuel. Many people don't understand that counting calories don't matter at this point since it is just used as a baseline.

Your body doesn't need glucose which will trigger these two stages:

- *The State of Glycogenesis*: The excess of glucose converts itself into glycogen, which is stored in the muscles and liver. Research indicates that only about half of your energy used daily can be saved as glycogen.

- *The State of Lipogenesis:* This phase is introduced when there is an adequate supply of glycogen in your liver and muscles, with any excess being converted to fat and stored.

Your body will have no more food (much like when you are sleeping), making your body burn the fat to create ketones. Once the ketones break down the fats, which generate fatty acids, they will burn-off in the liver through beta-oxidation. Thus, when you no longer have a supply of glycogen or glucose, ketosis begins and will use the consumed/stored fat as energy.

When the glycerol and fatty acid molecules are released, the ketogenesis process begins, and acetoacetate is produced. The Acetoacetate is converted to two types of ketone units:

- *Acetone:* This is mostly excreted as waste but can also be metabolized into glucose. This is the reason individuals on a ketogenic diet will experience a distinctive smelly breath.

- *Beta-Hydroxybutyrate or BHB:* Your muscles will convert the acetoacetate into BHB, which will fuel your brain after you have been on the keto diet for a short time.

You will discover how flexible the ketogenic methods are once you have all of the essential staples in your cabinets and fridge. Just remember, everyone will lose weight differently, and other people may not have the same goals as you.

For now, as a beginner, you will begin by using the first method, as shown below. This is an important step; you must decide how you want to proceed with your diet plan. It is always best to discuss this essential step with your physician. These are the four methods, so you better understand the different levels of the keto diet plan:

*Keto Technique 1:* The standard ketogenic diet (SKD) consists of moderate protein, high-fat, and is low in carbs. Generally, this diet is considered a low-carbohydrate (5% average), high-fat (75% average), and moderate protein (20%) diet plan. These are average counts and can vary.

*Keto Technique 2:* Workout times will call for the targeted keto diet, which is also called TKD. The process consists of adding additional carbohydrates to the diet plan during the times when you are more active. This is popular with sportsmen and women who are much more active.

*Keto Technique 3:* The cyclical ketogenic diet (CKD) entails a restricted five-day keto diet plan followed by two high-carbohydrate days.

*Keto Technique 4:* The high-protein keto diet is comparable to the standard keto plan (SKD) in all aspects. You will consume more protein. Its ratio is repeatedly noted as maintaining 35% protein, 5% carbs, and 60% fat. (Once again, these are average percentages.)

The Internet provides you with several ways to calculate your daily intake of carbs. Try a keto calculator to assist you. Begin your weight loss process by making a habit of checking your levels when you want to know what essentials your body needs during your dieting plan. You will document your personal information, such as height and weight. The Internet calculator will provide you with essential math.

# Chapter 1: Overview of the Keto Diet

Everywhere you look, there are so-called dietary experts that claim to know the secrets of the human body. They claim to have the secrets that can lead to sustained weight loss while guaranteeing that pounds will stay off permanently. However, many of these self-proclaimed gurus lack the fundamental knowledge that can enable their followers to truly gain the most out of the diets they promote. That is why this chapter is dedicated to revealing the inner workings of the keto diet, what it is, and what it is not.

The keto diet boils down to a low carb, high fat diet in which processed foods and refined carbs are to be reduced down to bare minimums. On the flipside, the keto diet calls for a greater consumption of fats, mainly good fats. Good fats are the kind which promote healthy energy production, efficient metabolism and most importantly, improved cognitive performance.

When looking at the keto diet, it is quite common to confuse it with the Atkins diet. The main difference with the Atkins diet is that the keto diets doesn't call for any specific restrictions on food. What it does call for is the restriction of cabs. This implies that you can virtually consume any type of food without overdoing the portion size.

Nevertheless, keto diet practitioners advocate and overall cleanup of a person's diet meaning the gradual elimination of processed foods while increasing the consumption of fresh fruits meats.

The textbook keto diet involves consuming fruits, vegetables and meats. Often, it is confused with going vegan or cutting out carbs altogether. While a vegan diet works well with the keto dietary approach, the fact of the matter is that cutting out carbs altogether can be detrimental to your health.

The main reason why carbs are important in a person's diet lies in the production of energy. When carbs enter the body, they are digested and subsequently converted into glucose. Glucose is one of the elements, along with oxygen, which the body uses to produce energy. As such, muscles burn glucose and oxygen in muscle tissue in order to power the body.

As long as the body is able to consume enough carbs and get enough oxygen intake, it will function as it was meant to. Things can get out of whack when the body doesn't get enough oxygen (which is rather unlikely) or there is an excess of glucose.

Therefore, having an excess of glucose in the bloodstream is problematic for the body as it needs to find a place to put it. The easiest thing the body can do to deal with excess glucose is convert it to fat and store it in between muscle tissue and the skin.

**Evolution plays a key role in fat storage**

The human body evolved under very harsh conditions. Early humans had by no means the access to food that we have today. In fact, early humans were quite likely to go days, even weeks, on very low caloric intake. This implied that they needed to make the most of the calories they consumed when they were able to.

In addition, our ancestors needed to live off the land. This implied knowing which plants were edible (a few surely died from eating poisonous plants) and being able to identify were they grew. Ideally, there would be a continuous supply of plants and fruits throughout the year. However, it is quite probable that most fruits and plants were not available year-round. So, this meant a rather limited supply of food.

As for animals, early hunters weren't always successful in catching fish or prey animals on a regular basis. So, when they were able to catch game, the meat would have been consumed along with the animal's fatty tissue. This is what provided early humans with the building blocks of the human body as we know it today.

The truth of the matter is that our diet is only about 60 years old. Since the end of World War II, food production has significantly increased throughout the world. As a result, Western cultures have had unprecedented access to food, the likes which had never been seen throughout human history.

Therefore, a diet that is high in carbs and sugar, and low in fat and protein, is essential the complete opposite from what our body was built on. It's kind of like loading up your car on water instead of gas and hoping it'll run just the same. Naturally, if your car was meant to run on gas, then water just won't work.

The same goes for the human body.

You need to give it the fuel it was designed to consume if you expect it to run as efficiently as it possibly can. Otherwise, you will encounter negative side effects, such as obesity and diabetes, when you load up on too much carb and saturated fats.

Now, it's important to note that this evolutionary response of the human body to carbs is rooted in its hardwiring. Since the body is hardwired to store as many calories as possible, it will do its best to accumulate as much fat as it possibly can.

Think about it based on the life early humans had. It only makes sense that the body would evolve this type of conditioning and reaction. After all, if you knew you wouldn't have access to food all the time, then you would do your best to store as much of it as you could.

The body does the same.

Under that premise, let's assume that your body overloads on calories, but then that caloric intake is reduced, then that gives the body a chance to process all that fat. However, if you keep a high amount of caloric intake on a consistent basis, the body has no choice but to get fat. This leads to obesity and obesity leads to any number of health issues.

**The keto diet and insulin resistance**

The keto diet is a great way to help the body process glucose. But, how does the body process glucose?

The body produces a hormone called "insulin". Insulin is used to process glucose and convert it to useful energy which the muscles and organ systems can utilize in their functioning. All of this works just fine so long as the body is not overloaded with glucose.

Insulin is primarily produced by the pancreas. The pancreas usually gets a break in between meals. This means that when a person eats, the pancreas secretes insulin, process foods and then takes a break until the next mealtime. This is one of the reasons why intermittent fasting tends to be beneficial specifically for people with diabetes.

The phenomenon known as "insulin resistance" occurs when there is so much glucose in the body that insulin production in insufficient to keep up with the amount of glucose circulating in the bloodstream. The situation worsens when cells essentially stop accepting glucose leaving glucose in the bloodstream with nowhere to go.

As a result, the keto diet helps people with insulin resistance get a better grip on the condition as it allows the body to process whatever amount of glucose is already in the body. This gives the body a chance to catch up while giving the pancreas and digestive system a break. When your body gets this break, it begins to progressively recover from the overload that it was once subjected to.

**The need for fat**

In recent time, fat has been vilified. And while fat is not necessarily a good thing, it depends on which type of fat we are talking about. The evil kind of fat creates cholesterol. Cholesterol then can lead to buildup in blood vessels eventually causing heart disease and associated illnesses. Needless to say, this is not a healthy way of living.

What most people fail to realize is that there is good cholesterol and bad cholesterol. Let's focus on bad cholesterol first.

Bad cholesterol is known as "LDL". LDL cholesterol is the kind that builds up in the arteries reducing the flow of blood in the body. In addition to causing circulatory problems, it can lead to increase risk of heart attack and stroke. Most folks go for years without noticing any symptoms of LDL until it is practically too late. By then, their risk of heart disease and stroke will have significantly increased.

LDL is generally the result of too much fat consumption, specifically saturated and trans fats. These are the types of fats that are produced as a result of fried foods. This is one of the reasons why "junk food" does a bad job on your body. During the frying process, oils and grease degrade into heavier fats which the body cannot digest. Since the body is able to virtually eliminate any unwanted substance, occasional consumption of bad fats won't produce any long-term effects on the body.

Things get complicated when there is a constant intake of these types of fats. Since the body is unable to get rid of them quickly enough, they begin to accumulate within blood vessels. The end result can be disastrous.

Do you see a pattern here?

The keto diet calls for the consumption of good fats which lead to the production of good cholesterol known as "HDL". Good cholesterol is useful for healthy hormone production. This creates a feedback loop which also helps the body produce enough insulin to keep up with carb intake. As a result, this promotes a cycle that leads to overall healthy living.

Healthy fats are found in fatty tissue in meat as well as plants and nuts such as avocados and brazil nuts. These are excellent sources of healthy fats which the body can easily digest and transform into HDL.

**The keto diet is rooted in evolution**

Based on the discussion we have presented in this chapter it is easy to see how the keto diet is rooted in the human body's natural evolution. It takes into account how early humans evolved under truly harsh conditions in which food wasn't always available. As a result, the keto diet looks to establish a dietary regimen that the body can utilize to ensure proper functioning.

Of course, it is entirely plausible that our bodies will eventually adapt to modern diets in which there is a higher amount of carb consumption. Perhaps the body will evolve in such a way that it will process carbs much more effectively and develop mechanisms in which it can reduce its tendency to store fat.

But the likelihood of these changes taking place in the short term are null. If anything, these are changes that take place over hundreds, if not thousands, of years. We may see these adaptations taking place over several generations.

In the meantime, we need to play to our body's strengths. That is why taking up the keto diet is nothing more than a logical step toward ensuring the body's natural functions. Consequently, you will be giving your body exactly what it needs. Thus, you will end up getting the benefits you seek.

# Chapter 2: The Benefits of the Keto Diet

The keto diet has a great deal of benefits that you can take advantage of. These benefits are generally associated to the proper functioning of the body while helping you deal with any conditions you may already be dealing with. As such, we will be focusing this chapter on the benefits you that come with taking on the keto diet.

## 1. Shedding unwanted pounds

Perhaps the main reason why most folks go on the keto diet is because they are looking to drop unwanted pounds. This is a perfectly logical reason to improve your diet especially since being overweight can lead to any number of health issues.

In addition to health issues, there is always the desire to look better and feel better about oneself. When folks have this kind of motivation, the keto diet can provide a solid alternative to losing weight and keeping it off.

There is one very important element to consider when going on the keto diet: it is important to reduce the consumption of processed foods. As stated earlier, the keto diet doesn't necessarily call for you to cut out processed foods or junk food altogether. What it does call for you is for you to reduce the consumption of these types of foods to an absolutely minimum. Ideally, you would be able to get rid of them for good.

When you consume enough carbs to fuel your lifestyle while increasing the amount of protein and healthy fats, you will be giving your metabolism the boost it needs to work at its optimal level. The end result will be a much more efficient metabolic process.

But there is one additional benefit: when the body is able to process carbs efficiently, it will invariably need to draw on its fat stores when there is an increased energetic requirement. For example, when you exercise, your body will need to increase its energy supply in order to keep up with the rate of the exercise you are doing. At this point, the body will have no choice but to draw on its fat reserves by converting back into glucose and burning them in muscle tissue.

This is how you can ensure fat burning and weight loss.

## 2. Hormone regulation

A common area which tends to give people trouble is proper hormone regulation. This occurs when a person's diet is heavy on carbs and light on fat and protein. Since the body doesn't have the building blocks it needs to repair itself, it tries to compensate in other areas. This leads the body prone to imbalances throughout each system. Consequently, finding the right balance is essential to helping the body find the right balance.

The hormone which suffers most in a high carb diet is insulin. As we have described earlier, insulin takes a huge hit when large amounts of glucose hit the bloodstream. Beyond insulin, other hormones such as testosterone and estrogen take a hit. The main reason for this is that male and female hormones rely on fat to reproduce themselves. Therefore, a diet that it low in fat will invariably lead to such types of imbalances.

But there is one hormone which creates nasty effects in the body: cortisol. Cortisol is secreted by the body whenever it undergoes a stress response. The function of cortisol is to send the body into a state of alert amid perceived danger. This state of alert heightens the immune system and sends blood pressure racing. Thus, it prepares the body for the fight or flight response.

When cortisol enters the bloodstream, it is meant to be discarded once the stress response is over. However, when there are hormonal imbalances, the body is unable to regulate itself back to normal. This implies that cortisol is not discarded by the body. Rather, it is reabsorbed and persists in circulation. When there is an excess of cortisol in the body, the most immediate effect is weight gain due to hoarding of fat. Please bear in mind that this is a stress response which prepares the body for the worst. The end result is weight gain, poor sleep regulation and premature aging.

Another hormone that goes off kilter is melatonin. Melatonin is the "sleep" hormone. This means that its absence does not allow the body to relax and get to sleep. When there is not enough melatonin production, the brain has trouble shutting down the nervous system. This is a good explanation as to why you may be terribly tired but unable to sleep. In the worst of cases, poor melatonin production can lead to insomnia which leads to further hormonal imbalances. As you can see, this turns out to be a vicious cycle which can be very hard to break.

In the end, the keto diet's call for restricting carb intake leads the body to normalize its functions thereby allowing for a good night's sleep, proper mood regulation and adequate metabolic function.

### 3. Improved cognitive ability

The brain is a power-hungry organ. The brain, and the nervous system by extension, consume the largest amount of energy. Given the fact that the nervous system runs the body's entire functions, there is a clear need for lots of energy.

When there are high amounts of the glucose in the body, the brain goes into overdrive. However, the brain itself cannot convert glucose into usable energy. This needs to happen as a result of the metabolic process that coverts oxygen and glucose into energy. Therefore, the brain shows massive spikes when there is considerable carb intake, and the sharp declines once the amount of glucose is reduced. This explains why sugar rushes ultimately lead to debilitating crashes. Caffeine has a similar effect on the brain.

When the body is running at an optimal level, the brain gets more usable energy and less glucose. This enables the brain to go about its business as it was designed for. By the same token, it is able to regulate it chemistry since it has the building blocks it needs to produce the right amount of hormones.

When the brain is running at its best possible level, there is a noticeable improvement in cognitive ability. Hence, the nervous system begins to regulate itself properly. For instance, if you had a tough day at the office, you may experience a spike in cortisol levels. Once the day is done, the brain will be able to regulate cortisol levels and ultimately produce enough melatonin to give you a good night's sleep.

In the case of students, the keto diet is perfect for enhancing overall cognitive ability. When the brain makes efficient use of its levels of energy, the run of the mill student can focus longer and study harder. The opposite effect is achieved when students gorge on sugar and caffeine. The brain gets the spike, but then crashes back down to levels inferior to those it began with.

## 4. Achieving ketosis

Ketosis is the state in which the metabolism is functioning at its optimal level. This is when there is the most efficient conversion of glucose into energy. By the same token, protein and fats are absorbed by the body in the possible manner.

However, ketosis is nearly impossible to achieve when there is high carb intake. This is another reason why the keto diet is quite adamant about reducing carb intake as much as possible. Again, this isn't about eliminating carb intake altogether; that is downright dangerous. The keto diet is about limiting the amount of carbs consumed so that the body has just enough to produce the energy it needs to power the body.

One of the most interesting effects of ketosis is the production of a substance known as ketones. Ketones are produced in liver as a result of the metabolic process that converts stored fat in the liver into usable energy that the brain can use to run the entire nervous system.

In fact, high levels of blood sugar lead to a condition known as "fatty liver". Fatty liver can be produced by drinking massive amount of alcohol, which is metabolized by the liver as glucose, and the consumption of large amounts of carbs and sugar. Thus, the keto diet also calls for the curtailing of alcohol. Generally speaking, alcohol should be consumed in small amounts though wine is much more acceptable as compared to other alcoholic beverages such as rum and beer which go straight into the bloodstream as glucose.

When the liver is no longer overwhelmed by the massive amounts of glucose it needs to metabolize, it can then use the fat it has in store and produce ketones. Ketones go straight into the brain and provide it with the energy it needs to manufacture hormones and regulate the nervous system. As you can see, achieving ketosis is the most significant improvement that stems from the keto diet.

### 5. Improved sleep

With the improvement of hormonal production and regulation, proper melatonin levels enable the brain to power down and get to sleep. But it's not just a question of getting to sleep, it's also a question of quality of sleep.

When the brain is unable to regulate the nervous system effectively, sleep patterns become altered as the brain is unable to calm down and enter the state known as "deep sleep". Deep sleep is a state in which the brain is able to enter a type of maintenance mode thus enabling it to repair the body and trigger proper hormonal regulation. Deep sleep occurs in 4-hour cycles meaning that even if you slept 4 hours only, you would still get better quality sleep than if you slept for 12 under poor quality sleep.

Deep sleep is also important for adequate regulation of glucose and insulin levels, production of good cholesterol and overall housekeeping. This housekeeping process is what allows the body to eliminate waste products and provide it with the elements it needs to sufficiently repair the body and ensure that all systems are fully operational.

It should also be noted that sleep deprivation, or simply poor-quality sleep, affects cortisol levels in the body. This link between lack of sleep and the body's inability to regulate cortisol explains why getting good quality sleep is essential in weight loss and enabling the body to achieve proper metabolic performance.

### 6.  Improved gut health

High carb intake is a known culprit of poor digestive health. Large amounts of carbs have been linked to poor gut health. By "poor gut health" we are referring to the inability of the body to produce the bacteria needed to process food appropriately. This, in turn, leads to poor absorption of nutrients such as vitamins and minerals. As such, a high carb diet would derail any attempts you made to improve your nutrition as your body would be unable to absorb the largest amount of nutrients.

Consider this situation: you are taking a vitamin supplement to fill the gaps of your nutrition. Moreover, your nutrition consists largely of carbs and meat while consuming low amounts of fat and plant-based protein. Sure, the supplement helps fill in the gaps in your nutrition, but the high amount of carbs does not allow the digestive system to absorb the nutrients contained in the supplement. In a manner of speaking, it's as if the glucose in the bloodstream blocked the doorway for any other type of nutrient to get through. Ultimately, there is very poor absorption of the nutrients needed for proper health and wellness.

There is one other reason why fat is so important in the keto diet. There are certain vitamins which are not soluble in water. Rather they are soluble in fact. This means that the body needs a certain amount of fat in order to process these vitamins and absorb them into the bloodstream. These vitamins include, A, D, E and K. Meanwhile, other vitamins such as B vitamins are soluble in water. That also means that if you don't drink enough water, your system cannot process them adequately.

When the body is unable to process fat-soluble vitamins, it simply discards them. Therefore, they are usually excreted in urine. So, even if you took a good vitamin supplement, or if you made sure to eat vitamin-rich foods, your body would be unable to absorb them properly until glucose levels come back down to normal. This can only be achieved when carb intake is reduced to adequate levels.

# Chapter 3: Getting Started with the Keto Diet

Thus far, we have extolled the benefits of the keto diet. We have presented the benefits and the most significant ways in which you overall health and wellbeing stand to reap the rewards of this dietary regimen.

However, most first-time keto diet practitioners may be unsure about how to get started. That is a perfectly reasonable concern as it's not always easy to change eating habits especially if you find yourself addicted to certain substances such as sugar.

That is why we are going to devote this chapter to laying out a transition process in which you can make the switch from your current eating habits, such as they are, into the keto diet approach.

Now, it should be noted that these changes don't happen overnight. In fact, the last thing you should be considering is giving up carbs and sugar overnight. First of all, it is unsustainable. This means that giving up sugar cold turkey will only lead you to binge when you simply are unable to control cravings. Thus, you can easily derail weeks of progress in one night of binge eating ice cream or pizza.

This is why it's always a good idea to gradually cut down on processed foods, sugar, alcohol, soft drinks and fried foods. As you gradually cut down, you will find that cravings become less and less predominant while giving yourself the chance to make healthier choice. In fact, the secret to making a successful transition lies in giving yourself the chance to make healthier choices.

Please bear in mind that making a drastic transition may trigger withdrawal symptoms in your body. These symptoms are essentially your body sending out an alert indicating that it is running low on a certain substance. For example, when you experience withdrawal symptoms after giving up sugar, you may feel nausea, headache, insatiable thirst and even dizzy spells. Other folks report feeling low levels or energy and even depression-like symptoms. Indeed, withdrawal is not an easy thing to deal with.

So, here are some guidelines which you can follow to help you make a smooth transition from your current diet to the keto diet.

### 1. Have clear goals

One of the goals you surely have in mind is losing weight. That is not only a reasonable goal but a necessary one. We have underscored several times the need for dropping pounds as obesity can lead to a series of health issues.

However, your weight loss goals need to be reasonable as well. You can't expect to lose 20 pounds in a month. This would not only be quite difficult to do, but quite unhealthy as it could lead the body to enter a state of shock.

So, set a reasonable target for yourself. Something like dropping 5 pounds in the first month is quite an achievement. In fact, most people don't lose a great deal of weight in the first few weeks. As a matter of fact, this is one of the reasons why some folks try the keto diet and give up on it. The truth is that it takes your body some time to eliminate the excessive levels of glucose and fat. When your body finally catches up to speed, it is then able to begin drawing from fat stores and weight loss occurs.

There is one caveat to weight loss. If you combine the keto diet with exercise including resistance exercises such as lifting weights, you may find that you won't "lose weight" but rather, you will lose "fat". This is an important distinction to make as the weight lost in terms of fat can be regained in terms of muscle. Naturally, this is a tradeoff you want to take every time.

## 2. Ease into it

Making changes of any kind can be complex. That is why easing into the keto diet is your best bet to make it stick. By "easing into it" we mean you ought to look at ways in which you can cut back on your carb consumption. For instance, if you find that you are eating take out virtually every night, you might want to think about cutting to two nights a week. The nights that you don't have takeout, you can plan any one of the recipe ideas we have provided in this book. Please bear in mind that making any sudden changes will render your attempt to switch to the keto diet that much harder to stick.

Also, it's a good idea to gradually cut back on soft drinks and alcoholic beverages. While we are not saying that they are entirely off-limits, we are saying that it's important to cut back on them as much as possible. In fact, you can set a quota. For example, if you go out with friends on a Saturday night, you can limit yourself to a couple of beers. That is much better than chugging down all you can drink.

### 3. Plan your meals

The biggest culprit of poor eating choices is lack of planning. When you don't plan your meals, you may find yourself struggling to figure out what to make for lunch or dinner. This is especially worrisome when you are pressed for time. For instance, when you are running late from work and you haven't had time to cook, opting for takeout is the easier route to go.

That's why we have included a sample 7-day plan for you to get a good idea of how you can plan your meals. This will allow you to find a good balance between yummy foods and a nutritious alternative. In the end, you will find the best of both worlds as you won't have to wrack your brain trying to figure out what to make for dinner. In fact, planning meals also saves money as you only purchase what you actually plan to eat.

### 4. Don't skip breakfast

There should be "wanted" posters for skipping breakfast. When you skip breakfast, you allow your body to become hungrier than it should. This almost always leads to binging on carbs as they tend to be the most filling and satisfying. This is why pizza tastes so good when you are really hungry.

So, make a point of having breakfast all the time. In this book, you will find easy and healthy options that won't carve a chunk out of your schedule. If anything, you can easily prepare these breakfast options even when you are running late.

By making sure that you don't skip out on breakfast, you will allow yourself to curb your hunger and avoid making poor food choices. Ultimately, this will be a big step toward achieving your ultimate goals.

## 5. Set a schedule

Another culprit of weight gain is eating at odd hours. This includes the occasional midnight snack. Now, there's nothing wrong with a snack. But when a snack becomes something closer to a meal, then it's a good idea to make sure that you have a schedule in mind.

A good rule of thumb is eating roughly 3 hours before your bedtime. So, if you plan to go to bed at 10, it is advisable to have dinner around 7. By the same token, you ought to consider having breakfast roughly one hour after getting up. Lunch time is up to you and entirely dependent on your schedule. Snacks should be placed roughly 2 to 3 hours after a meal. In fact, you might find that some dietary experts recommend that you eat every four hours. This advice is consistent with the amount of time the metabolism needs to reset after each meal.

Furthermore, a rather consistent schedule will help your metabolism establish a game plan. That way, your body knows when it's time to eat and when it's time to rest. Make sure that you leave a proper amount of time between meals. That will give your digestive system the time it needs to rest and prepare for the next meal.

# Chapter 4: Breakfast & Brunch Recipe Ideas

## Asiago Bagels

**Servings**: 8

**Nutritional Facts Per Serving**:

- Protein Counts: 20 g

- Total Fats: 21 g

- Calories: 293

- Net Carbohydrates: 6 g

**Ingredients:**

- Almond flour (1.5 cups/192 g)

- Eggs (2)

- Gluten-free baking powder (1 tbsp.)

- Sea salt (.5 tsp.)

- Shredded mozzarella (2 cups/256 g)

- Cream cheese (.25 cup/32 g)

- Shredded asiago (1 cup/128 g)

## Preparation Technique:

1. Set the oven setting at 400F/205C.

2. Combine the salt, almond flour, eggs, and baking powder.

3. In a microwave-safe container, melt the mozzarella and cream cheese. Mix the melted mixture, almond flour mixture, with 3/4 cup/96 g of shredded asiago.

4. Shape into a ball and knead until each of the fixings is thoroughly combined. Break the dough into eight pieces and shape each ball into bagel forms.

5. Sprinkle the remaining 1/4 cup/32 g of asiago cheese onto the bagels. Arrange on a baking tray to bake for about 20 minutes.

# Bacon & Avocado Omelet

**Servings**: 1

**Nutritional Facts Per Serving**:

- Protein Counts: 30 g

- Total Fats: 63 g

- Calories: 719

- Net Carbohydrates: 3.3 g

**Ingredients:**

- Crispy bacon (1 slice)

- Large organic eggs (2)

- Freshly grated parmesan cheese (.5 cup/64 g)

- Ghee or coconut oil or butter (2 tbsp.)

- Avocado (half of 1 small)

**Preparation Steps:**

1. Prepare the bacon to your liking and set it aside.

2. Combine the eggs, parmesan cheese, and your choice of finely chopped herbs.

3. Warm a skillet and add the butter/ghee to melt using the medium-high heat setting.

4.  When the pan is hot, whisk and add the eggs.

5.  Prepare the omelet working it towards the middle of the pan for about 30 seconds. When firm, flip, and cook it for another 30 seconds.

6.  Arrange the omelet on a plate and garnish with the crunched bacon bits. Serve with sliced avocado.

# Bacon - Egg & Cheese Cups

**Servings**: 6

**Nutritional Facts Per Serving**:

- Protein Counts: 8 g

- Total Fats: 7 g

- Calories: 101

- Net Carbohydrates: 1 g

**Ingredients:**

- Bacon (6 strips)

- Large eggs (6)

- Cheese (.25 cup/32 g)

- Fresh spinach (1 handful)

- Pepper (as desired)

**Preparation Technique:**

1. Set the oven setting to 400F/204C.

2. Prepare the bacon using medium heat on the stovetop. Place it on towels to drain.

3. Grease six muffin tins with a spritz of oil. Line each tin with a slice of bacon, pressing tightly to make a secure well for the eggs.

4. Drain and dry the spinach with a paper towel. Whisk the eggs and combine with the spinach.

5. Add the mixture to the prepared tins and sprinkle with cheese. Sprinkle with salt and pepper until it's like you like it.

6. Bake for 15 minutes. Remove when done and serve or cool to store in the fridge.

# Bacon & Cheese Frittata

**Servings: 6**

**Nutritional Facts Per Serving:**

- Protein Counts: 13 g

- Total Fats: 29 g

- Calories: 320

- Net Carbohydrates: 2 g

**Ingredients:**

- Heavy cream (1 cup/128 g)

- Eggs (6)

- Black pepper (.25 tsp.)

- Salt (.5 tsp.)

- Heavy cream (1 cup/ 128g)

- Crispy bacon (5 slices)

- Green onions (2)

- Cheddar cheese (4 oz./ 115 g)

- Also Needed: 1 pie plate

**Preparation Technique:**

1. Set the oven temperature to 350F/175C.

2.  Chop the onions and cook the bacon until it's crispy.

3.  Whisk the eggs and seasonings. Empty them into the pie pan and top it off with the rest of the fixings.

4.  Bake 30 to 35 minutes. Wait for a few minutes before serving for the best results.

# Bacon & Egg Muffins

**Servings**: 12

**Nutritional Facts Per Serving**:

- Protein Counts: 5.6 g

- Total Fats: 4.9 g

- Calories: 69

- Net Carbohydrates: 0.4 g

**Ingredients**:

- Eggs (8 large)

- Bacon (8 slices)

- Green onion (.66 cup/100 g)

**Preparation Technique:**

1. Warm the oven at 350F/177C. Spritz the muffin tin wells using a cooking oil spray. Chop the onions and set aside.

2. Prepare a large skillet using the medium temperature setting. Fry the bacon until it's crispy and place on a layer of paper towels to drain the grease. Chop it into small pieces after it has cooled.

3. Whisk the eggs, bacon, and green onions, mixing well until all of the fixings are incorporated.

4. Dump the egg mixture into the muffin tin (halfway full).

5. Bake it for about 20 to 25 minutes. Cool slightly and serve.

# Bagels & Cheese

**Servings**: 6

**Nutritional Facts Per Serving**:

- Protein Counts: 19 g

- Total Fats: 31 g

- Calories: 374

- Net Carbohydrates: 8 g

**Ingredients**:

- Mozzarella cheese (2.5 cups/282 g)

- Baking powder (1 tsp.)

- Cream cheese (3 oz./80 g)

- Almond flour (1.5 cups/144 g)

- Eggs (2)

**Preparation Technique:**

1. Shred the mozzarella and combine with the flour, baking powder, and cream cheese in a mixing container. Pop it into the microwave for about one minute, stirring well.

2. Let the mixture cool and add the eggs. Break the mixture apart into six sections and shape into round bagels.

3. *Note*: You can also sprinkle with a seasoning of your choice or pinch of salt if desired.

4. Bake them for approximately 12 to 15 minutes. Serve or cool and store.

# Banana Pancakes

**Servings**: 3

**Nutritional Facts Per Serving**:

- Total Fats: 7 g

- Calories: 157

- Net Carbohydrates: 6.8 g

**Ingredients**:

- Butter (as needed)

- Bananas (2)

- Eggs (4)

- Cinnamon (1 tsp.)

- Optional: Baking powder (.5 tsp.)

**Preparation Technique:**

1. Combine each of the fixings.

2. Melt a portion of butter in a skillet using the medium temperature setting.

3. Prepare the pancakes 1-2 minutes per side. Cook them with the lid on for the first part of the cooking cycle for a fluffier pancake.

4.

5.  Serve plain or with your favorite garnishes such as a dollop of coconut cream or fresh berries.

# Biscuits & Gravy

**Servings**: 2

**Nutritional Facts Per Serving**:

- Protein Counts: 22 g

- Total Fats: 36 g

- Calories: 425

- Net Carbohydrates: 2 g

**Ingredients**:

- Salt (.25 tsp.)

- Almond flour (.25 cup/24 g)

- Baking powder (.5 tsp.)

- Large egg white (1)

- Crumbled breakfast sausage (6 oz. pkg./ 170 g)

- Chicken broth (.25 cup/60 g)

- Cream cheese (.25 cup/55 g)

- Pepper and salt (to your liking)

**Preparation Technique**:

1. Set the oven at 400F/205C. Prepare a baking tin with a layer of parchment baking paper.

2. Whisk the salt, almond flour, and baking powder.

3. In another dish, whisk the egg whites to form stiff peaks.

4. Dice the butter into small pieces. Form a crumbled mixture in the dry components using the butter. Gently blend it into the egg whites.

5. Split the mixture into two portions on the paper-lined pan.

6. Bake for 11-15 minutes.

7. Using the medium heat setting, warm the sausage. When browned, add the cream cheese, chicken broth, pepper, and salt.

8. Serve with biscuits with a serving of the delicious gravy.

9. Prep time is only 15 minutes with a cooking time of only 25 minutes.

# BLT Wrap

**Servings**: 4

**Nutritional Facts Per Serving**:

- Protein Counts: 8 g

- Total Fats: 24 g

- Calories: 256

- Net Carbohydrates: 2 g

**Ingredients**:

- Crispy fried bacon slices (4)

- Romaine or Iceberg lettuce leaves (2)

- Chopped tomatoes (.25 cup/50 g)

- Mayo (1 tbsp.)

- Optional: Pepper

**Preparation Technique:**

1. Cook the bacon until crispy in a skillet or the microwave (your choice).

2. Spread a layer of mayonnaise on one side of the lettuce.

3. Add the bacon and tomato. Season the wrap to your liking. Roll it up and serve.

# Blueberry Scones

**Servings**: 12

**Nutritional Facts Per Serving**:

- Protein Counts: 2 g

- Total Fats: 8 g

- Calories: 133

- Net Carbohydrates: 4 g

**Ingredients**:

- Baking powder (2 tsp.)

- Almond flour (1.5 cups/144 g)

- Stevia (.5 cup/101 g)

- Vanilla (2 tsp.)

- Raspberries (.75 cup/95 g)

- Eggs (3)

**Preparation Technique:**

1. Warm up the oven to 375F/191C. Prepare a baking pan with a piece of parchment paper.

2. Whisk the baking powder, stevia, flour, and vanilla. Whisk the egg and add it to the mixture. Fold in the raspberries.

3.  Add the batter to the prepared baking sheet and place in the oven.

4.  Set a timer and bake them for 15 minutes. Remove the scones from the oven.

5.  Cool slightly before serving.

# Breakfast Burrito

**Servings**: 1

**Nutritional Facts Per Serving**:

- Protein Counts: 11 g
- Total Fats: 30 g
- Calories: 331
- Net Carbohydrates: 1 g

**Ingredients**:

- Butter (1 tbsp.)
- Medium eggs (2)
- Full-fat cream (2 tbsp.)
- Spices/herbs
- Pepper and salt (to your liking)

**Preparation Technique:**

1. Whisk the eggs and herbs/spices in a mixing container.

2. Prepare a skillet with butter and add the burrito mixture. Swirl it in the pan. Cover and cook for two minutes.

3. Serve the burrito right out of the pan!

# Brunch Zucchini Bread - Slow-Cooked

**Servings**: 12 slices

**Nutritional Facts Per Serving**:

- Protein Counts: 5 g

- Total Fats: 15.7 g

- Calories: 174

- Net Carbohydrates: 13.8 g

**Ingredients**:

- Almond flour (1 cup/112 g)

- Cinnamon (2 tsp.)

- Coconut flour (.33 cup/40 g)

- Baking powder (1.5 tsp.)

- Optional: Xanthan gum (.5 tsp.)

- Salt (.5 tsp.)

- Baking soda (.5 tsp.)

- Softened coconut oil or butter (.33 cup/73 g)

- Eggs (3)

- Vanilla (2 tsp.)

- Pyure all-purpose (.5 cup/182 g)

- Shredded zucchini (2 cups/248 g)

- Chopped pecans or walnuts (.5 cup/59 g)

- Also Needed: 4x8 silicone bread pan

**Preparation Technique:**

1. Combine the coconut and almond flour, salt, baking soda, and powder, cinnamon, and xanthan gum. Set aside for now.

2. Mix the oil, eggs, vanilla, and sugar in another dish. Combine the fixings.

3. Blend in the nuts and shredded zucchini. Scoop the batter into the prepared bread pan.

4. Arrange the cooker on the top rack (or on crunched up aluminum foil balls). You want it at least 1/2-inch from the bottom of the slow cooker.

5. Put the top onto the cooker and prepare for three hours using the high-temperature setting.

6. Cool, wrap in foil, and place in the fridge. It is best when refrigerated.

# Butter Coffee

**Servings**: 1

**Nutritional Facts Per Serving**:

- Protein Counts: 0 g

- Total Fats: 25 g

- Calories: 230

- Net Carbohydrates: 0 g

**Ingredients**:

- Coffee (2 tbsp.)

- Grass-fed butter (1 tbsp.)

- Water (1 cup/236 g)

- Coconut oil (1 tbsp.)

**Preparation Technique:**

1. Prepare your favorite cup of coffee. Combine the brewed coffee, butter, and coconut in a blender.

2. Puree it for about 10 seconds until it's light in color and creamy. Enjoy for breakfast when you are in a hurry or anytime for a refreshing treat.

# Cheesy Mushroom Omelet

**Servings**: 1

**Nutritional Facts Per Serving**:

- Protein Counts: 25 g

- Total Fats: 43 g

- Calories: 510

- Net Carbohydrates: 4 g

**Ingredients**:

- Butter (1 oz./28 g)

- Eggs (3)

- Shredded cheese (1 oz./28 g)

- Yellow onion (3 tbsp.)

- Mushrooms (3)

- Pepper and Salt (to your liking)

**Preparation Technique:**

1. Add the butter to a skillet.

2. Whisk the eggs, spices, salt, and pepper until frothy.

3. Prepare the omelet. Once the bottom is firm, sprinkle in the onions, mushrooms, and cheese.

4.  Carefully remove the edges and fold the omelet in half.

5.  Slide onto a plate when it's done.

# Choco-Breakfast Waffles

**Servings**: 5

**Nutritional Facts Per Serving**:

- Protein Counts: 7 g

- Total Fats: 27 g

- Calories: 289

- Net Carbohydrates: 3.4 g

**Ingredients**:

- Separated eggs (5)

- Unsweetened cocoa (.25 cup/30 g)

- Granular sweetener (3 tbsp.)

- Coconut flour (4 tbsp.)

- Baking powder (1 tsp.)

- Melted butter (4.5 oz./130 g)

- Milk of choice (3 tbsp.)

- Vanilla (1 tsp.)

**Preparation Technique:**

1. Break the eggs into a mixing bowl and whisk the egg whites briskly to form stiff peaks.

2.  In another container, whisk the sweetener, baking powder, cocoa, with the egg yolks.

3.  Slowly, add the butter to the dry mixture. Stir in the vanilla and milk.

4.  Fold in the prepared egg whites a little at a time.

5.  Transfer the mixture in the waffle maker and cook until they are golden brown.

# Coconut-Almond Egg Wraps

**Servings**: 4

**Nutritional Facts Per Serving**:

- Protein Counts: 8 g

- Total Fats: 8 g

- Calories: 111

- Net Carbohydrates: 3 g

**Ingredients**:

- Eggs (5)

- Coconut flour (1 tbsp.)

- Sea salt (.25 tsp.)

- Almond meal (2 tbsp.)

**Preparation Technique:**

1. Combine the fixings in a blender and work them until creamy.

2. Heat a skillet using the med-high temperature setting.

3. Pour two tablespoons of batter into the skillet and cook - covered about three minutes.

4.  Turn it over to cook for another 3 minutes.

5.  Serve the wraps piping hot.

53

# Coffee Cake

**Servings**: 8

**Nutritional Facts Per Serving**:

- Protein Counts: 13 g

- Total Fats: 28 g

- Calories: 321

- Net Carbohydrates: 4 g

**Ingredients**:

*For The Base:*

- Eggs (6 separated)

- Cream cheese (6 oz./170 g)

- Erythritol (.25 cup/25 g)

- Liquid stevia (.25 tsp.)

- Unflavored protein powder (.25 cup/25 g)

- Cream of tartar (.25 tsp.)

- Vanilla extract (2 tsp.)

*The Filling:*

- Cinnamon (1 tbsp.)

- Almond flour (1.5 cups/144 g)

- Butter (.5 stick)

- Maple Syrup Substitute (.25 cup/36 g)

- Erythritol (.25 cup/45 g)

- Also Needed: Dark metal cake pan

**Preparation Technique:**

1. Warm up the oven to 325F/163C.

2. Gently separate the egg whites from the yolks.

3. Whisk the egg yolks with the erythritol and add with the rest of the fixings. (Omit the egg whites and cream of tartar for the next step.)

4. Whisk the tartar and whites of the eggs to create stiff peaks. Gently work into the yolks.

5. Mix all of the filling fixings to form the dough.

6. Scoop the batter base into the pan. Top it off with ½ of the cinnamon - filling, pushing it down if needed.

7. Bake for 20 minutes. Transfer to the countertop.

8. Prepare the cake with the rest of the filling dough.

9. Bake for another 20 minutes to half an hour.

10. Cool for 10 to 20 minutes before serving.

# Cream Cheese Eggs

**Servings**: 1

**Nutritional Facts Per Serving**:

- Protein Counts: 15 g

- Total Fats: 31 g

- Calories: 341

- Net Carbohydrates: 3 g

**Ingredients**:

- Butter (1 tbsp.)

- Eggs (2)

- Soft cream cheese with chives (2 tbsp.)

**Preparation Technique:**

1. Preheat a skillet and melt the butter.

2. Whisk the eggs with the cream cheese.

3. Add to the pan and stir until done.

# Healthy Bacon Hash & Eggs

**Servings**: 2

**Nutritional Facts Per Serving**:

- Protein Counts: 23 g

- Total Fats: 24 g

- Calories: 366

- Net Carbohydrates: 9 g

**Ingredients**:

- Bacon (6 slices)

- Small green pepper (1)

- Jalapenos (2)

- Small onion (1)

- Eggs (4)

**Preparation Technique:**

1. Chop the bacon into chunks using a food processor. Set it aside for now.

2. Slice the peppers and onions into thin strips and dice the jalapenos as small as possible.

3. Heat a skillet and fry the vegetables.

4. Once it's browned, combine the fixings and cook until
   crispy.

5. Place on a plate with the eggs.

# Italian Cheesy Omelet

**Servings**: 2

**Nutritional Facts Per Serving**:

- Protein Counts: 33 g

- Total Fats: 36 g

- Calories: 451

- Net Carbohydrates: 3 g

**Ingredients**:

- Eggs (2)

- Water (1 tbsp.)

- Butter or ghee (1 tbsp.)

- Salami or prosciutto (3 thin slices)

- Basil (6 leaves)

- Mozzarella cheese slices (2 oz./56 g)

- Tomato (5 thin slices)

- Pepper and salt (as desired)

**Preparation Technique:**

1. Toss the ghee/butter into a skillet (med. heat setting) to melt. Whisk the water and eggs together. Pour them

into the skillet to cook for about 30 seconds.

2.  Spread out the meat slices over top of the egg, followed by the cheese, slices of tomatoes, basil, pepper, and salt.

3.  Cook for approximately two minutes until firm. Flip, and continue cooking for another minute before folding in half. Simmer using low heat (top on).

4.  When the center is done, just add the omelet to a plate and serve.

# Mackerel & Eggs

**Servings**: 2

**Nutritional Facts Per Serving**:

- Protein Counts: 35 g

- Total Fats: 59g

- Calories: 4

- Net Carbohydrates: 4 g

**Ingredients**:

- Butter for frying (2 tbsp.)

- Eggs (4)

- Canned mackerel in tomato sauce (8 oz./226 g)

- Lettuce (2 oz./55 g)

- Red onion (half of 1)

- Olive oil (.25 cup/55 g)

- Black pepper & salt (to your liking)

**Preparation Technique:**

1. Warm the frying pan and prepare the eggs in the butter.

2. Add lettuce to a platter and layer with onion and

mackerel.

3. Arrange the eggs to the side, seasoning as desired using the pepper and salt.

4. Spritz the oil over the salad and serve.

# 1-Minute Keto Muffins

**Servings**: 1

**Nutritional Facts Per Serving**:

- Protein Counts: 7 g

- Total Fats: 6 g

- Calories: 113

- Net Carbohydrates: 2 g

**Ingredients**:

- Egg (1)

- Salt (a pinch)

- Coconut flour (2 tsp.)

- Baking soda (1 pinch)

- Butter/coconut oil (as needed)

**Preparation Technique:**

1. Lightly grease a large coffee mug/ramekin dish using butter or coconut

   oil/butter.

2. Whisk all of the fixings together and cook for one minute using high for 45 seconds to one minute in the microwave. You can also bake for 12 minutes at

400F/205C the oven.

3.  Slice in half or toast and serve.

# Sesame - Poppy Seed Bagels

**Servings**: 6

**Nutritional Facts Per Serving**:

- Protein Counts: 20 g

- Total Fats: 29 g

- Calories: 350

- Net Carbohydrates: 5 g

**Ingredients**:

- Sesame cheese (8 tsp.)

- Poppy seeds (8 tsp.)

- Shredded mozzarella cheese (2.5 cups/282 g)

- Baking powder (1 tsp.)

- Almond flour (1.5 cups/144 g)

- Large eggs (2)

**Preparation Technique:**

1. Set the oven at 400F/205C.

2. Prepare a baking pan using a layer of parchment paper. Sift the baking powder and flour.

3. Melt the cream cheese and mozzarella in a microwave-

safe dish for one minute. Stir and cook one more minute.

4. Whisk the eggs and add the cheese mixture with the rest of the fixings. Once the dough is formed, break it apart into six pieces.

5. Stretch the dough and join the ends to shape the bagels. Arrange on the baking tray.

6. Sprinkle with the seed combination and set a timer to bake for 15 minutes.

# Chapter 5: Lunchtime Favorites

## Avocado - Tuna Melt Bites

**Servings**: 12

**Nutritional Facts Per Serving**:

- Protein Counts: 5 g

- Total Fats: 17.8 g

- Calories: 185

- Net Carbohydrates: 1.02 g

**Ingredients**:

- Mayonnaise (.25 cup/57 g)

- Parmesan cheese (.25 cup/25 g)

- Drained tuna (10 oz./283 g)

- Almond flour (.33 cup/32 g)

- Onion powder (.25 tsp.)

- Garlic powder (.5 tsp.)

- Pepper and salt (to your liking)

- Cubed avocado (1 medium)

- Coconut oil for cooking (2 tbsp.)

**Preparation Technique:**

1. Prepare the avocado by removing the pit. Cut it into cubes.

2. Combine each of the fixings (omitting the oil and avocado).

3. Fold in the tuna with the avocado and shape into balls. Coat with flour.

4. Heat the oil using the medium temperature setting and fry until browned. Serve or store when it's cooled.

# Baked Zucchini Noodles with Feta

**Servings**:  3

**Nutritional Facts Per Serving**:

- Protein Counts: 4 g

- Total Fats: 8 g

- Calories: 105

- Net Carbohydrates: 5 g

**Ingredients**:

- Quartered plum tomato (1)

- Spiralized zucchini (2)

- Feta cheese (8 cubes)

- Pepper and salt (1 tsp. each)

- Olive oil (1 tbsp.)

**Preparation Technique:**

1. Lightly grease a roasting pan with a spritz of olive oil.

2. Warm the oven temperature to reach 375F/191C.

3. Slice the noodles with a spiralizer and add to the prepared pan along with the oil, salt, pepper, and tomatoes.

4. Bake it for 10 to 15 minutes. Transfer from the oven and add the cheese cubes, tossing to combine before serving.

# Ham & Spinach Mini Quiche

**Servings**: 2

**Nutritional Facts Per Serving**:

- Protein Counts: 20 g

- Total Fats: 13 g

- Calories: 210

- Net Carbohydrates: 2 g

**Ingredients**:

- Diced ham (4 slices)

- Whisked eggs (3)

- Chopped spinach (.75 cup/170 g)

- Chopped leek (.25 cup/25 g)

- Coconut milk (.25 cup/57 g)

- Baking powder (.5 tsp.)

- Pepper & salt (as desired)

**Preparation Technique:**

1. Warm up the oven temperature to 350F/177C.

2. Combine all of the fixings in a large mixing container.

3. Pour the mixture into tart pans or four small mini quiche pans.

4. Bake 15 minutes. Serve.

# Tuna Salad & Chives

**Servings**: 4

**Nutritional Facts Per Serving**:

- Protein Counts: 20 g

- Total Fats: 18 g

- Calories: 235

- Net Carbohydrates: 1 g

**Ingredients**:

- Tuna - packed in olive oil (15 oz./425 g)

- Mayonnaise (6 tbsp.)

- Chives (2 tbsp.)

- Pepper (.25 tsp.)

**Preparation Technique:**

1. Drain the tuna and finely chop the chives.

2. Add all of the fixings except the lettuce into a mixing bowl.

3. Toss well. Enjoy as-is or spoon into romaine lettuce leaves.

# Tuna Stuffed Avocado

**Servings**: 1

**Nutritional Facts Per Serving**:

- Protein Counts: 31 g

- Total Fats: 45 g

- Calories: 565

- Net Carbohydrates: 3 g

**Ingredients**:

- Greek yogurt/mayonnaise (2 tbsp.)

- Drained tuna (5 oz. can/141 g)

- Medium avocado (1)

- Dried dill (1 pinch)

**Preparation Technique:**

1. Combine the fixings (mayo, tuna, and dill).

2. Cut the avocado in half and remove the pit. Fill it with the salad and serve.

# Avocado - Corn Salad

**Servings**: 4

**Nutritional Facts Per Serving**:

- Protein Counts: 3.5 g

- Total Fats: 11 g

- Calories: 147

- Net Carbohydrates: 4.5 g

**Ingredients**:

*The Salad:*

- Cooked - corn on the cob - husk removed (1)

- Romaine head (1 chopped)

- Quartered grape tomatoes (4)

- Sliced red onion (.25 cup/25 g)

- Sliced avocado (half of 1)

*The Dressing:*

- Minced shallots (1 tbsp.)

- Dijon mustard (2 tsp.)

- 1% Vegan buttermilk (6 tbsp.)

- Garlic powder (.25 tsp.)

- Black pepper (1 pinch)

- Kosher salt (.5 tsp.)

- White wine vinegar (2 tbsp.)

- Extra-Virgin olive oil (2 tbsp.)

## Preparation Technique:

1. Whisk each of the dressing fixings and pour it into a serving jar.

2. Prepare and add the salad fixings in a large salad bowl. Toss it with the dressing.

# Caprese Salad

**Servings**: 4

**Nutritional Facts Per Serving**:

- Protein Counts: 7.7 g

- Total Fats: 63.5 g

- Calories: 191

- Net Carbohydrates: 4.6 g

**Ingredients**:

- Grape tomatoes (3 cups/600 g)

- Peeled garlic cloves (4)

- Avocado oil (2 tbsp.)

- Mozzarella balls (19 pearl-sized)

- Baby spinach leaves (4 cups/900 g)

- Fresh basil leaves (.25 cup/55 g)

- Brine reserved from the cheese (1 tbsp.)

- Pesto (1 tbsp.)

**Preparation Technique:**

1. Use a sheet of aluminum foil to cover a baking tray.

2. Set the oven temperature setting to 400F/204C.

3. Arrange the cloves and tomatoes on the baking pan and drizzle with oil. Bake for 20 to 30 minutes until the tops are lightly browned.

4. Drain the liquid (saving one tablespoon) from the mozzarella. Mix the pesto with the brine.

5. Arrange the spinach in a large serving bowl. Transfer the tomatoes to the dish along with the roasted garlic. Drizzle with the pesto sauce.

6. Garnish with the mozzarella balls and freshly torn basil leaves.

# Cobb Salad

**Servings**: 1

**Nutritional Facts Per Serving**:

- Protein Counts: 38.4 g

- Total Fats: 23.6 g

- Calories: 412

- Net Carbohydrates: 3.9 g

**Ingredients**:

- Cherry tomatoes (4)

- Avocado (half of 1)

- Hard-boiled egg (1)

- Mixed green salad (2 cups/150 g)

- Feta cheese - crumbled (1 oz./28 g)

- Chicken breast - shredded (2 oz./28 g)

- Cooked bacon - crumbled (.25 cup/55 g raw)

**Preparation Technique:**

1. Dice the tomatoes and avocado and slice a hard-boiled egg.

2. Toss the mixed green salad into a large salad bowl.

3. Measure out the shredded chicken breast, cheese, and crumbled bacon.

4. Add the avocado, tomatoes, chicken, egg, bacon, and feta in rows on top of the salad greens.

# Deviled Chicken Salad Eggs

**Servings**: 6

**Nutritional Facts Per Serving**:

- Protein Counts: 13 g

- Total Fats: 7 g

- Calories: 128

- Net Carbohydrates: 2 g

**Ingredients**:

- Old Bay Seasoning (1 dash/5 g)

- Lemon pepper (.5 tsp.)

- Dill (.5 tsp.)

- Celery salt (1 pinch)

- Chopped onion (1 tbsp.)

- Dijon mustard (1 tsp.)

- Mayonnaise (2 tbsp.)

- Shredded chicken (1 cup/125 g)

- Large eggs (6)

## Preparation Technique:

1. Combine all of the fixings, omit the eggs, and store in the fridge for later.

2. Gently place the eggs in a pot of water (just enough to cover the eggs).

3. Set the temperature on high until it boils and lower the setting to medium.

4. Boil for 15 minutes and transfer to cool under cold running water.

5. Remove the shell and slice the eggs into halves. Remove the yolk and fill with the salad mixture. Sprinkle with the old bay seasoning and serve.

6. *Note*: Discard the yolks or use them in another recipe. The total time is 30 minutes.

# Kale Parmesan Salad

**Servings**: 4

**Nutritional Facts Per Serving**:

- Protein Counts: 4 g

- Total Fats: 6 g

- Calories: 80

- Net Carbohydrates: 3 g

**Ingredients**:

- Salt (.5 tsp.)

- Olive oil (1 tbsp.)

- Kale (1 bunch)

- Lemon juice (1 tbsp.)

- Parmesan cheese (.33 cup/42 g)

**Preparation Technique:**

1. Remove the ribs from the kale and slice into ¼-inch strips.

2. Combine with the salt and oil, toss about 3 minutes until softened.

3. Toss the cheese, juice, and kale. Serve.

# Keto Salad Niçoise

**Servings**: 1

**Nutritional Facts Per Serving**:

- Protein Counts: 18 g

- Total Fats: 48 g

- Calories: 544

- Net Carbohydrates: 8 g

**Ingredients**:

- Large egg (1)

- Celery (.5 cup/115 g)

- Snow peas (.5 cup/75 g)

- Olive oil (2 tbsp.)

- Garlic (.25 tbsp.)

- Romaine lettuce (1 cup/75 g)

- Green onion (.5 tbsp.)

- Olives (.5 tbsp.)

- Crumbled feta cheese (.5 cup/75 g)

- Balsamic vinegar (1 tbsp.)

**Preparation Technique:**

1. Hard boil the egg and remove the peel when it's cooled.

2. Chop the garlic, onion, celery, and olives.

3. Pour the oil into a small pan. Sauté the garlic, olives, and snow peas until the peas are bright green.

4. Prepare a large salad dish and add the shredded lettuce, celery, cooked veggies, and green onion.

5. Make the dressing by whisking the vinegar, oil, salt, and pepper.

6. Combine the fixings and toss well before serving.

# Lobster Salad

**Servings**: 4

**Nutritional Facts Per Serving**:

- Protein Counts: 18 g

- Total Fats: 25 g

- Calories: 307

- Net Carbohydrates: 2 g

**Ingredients**:

- Melted butter (.25 cup/240 g)

- Cooked lobster meat (1 lb./453 g)

- Mayonnaise (.25 cup/57 g)

- Black pepper (.125 tsp.)

**Preparation Technique:**

1. Chop the lobster into bite-sized pieces.

2. Melt and pour the butter over the meat. Toss to coat and blend in the mayonnaise along with the pepper.

3. Chill in a covered dish for a minimum of 10 minutes or chilled to your liking.

# Steak Salad

**Servings**: 2

**Nutritional Facts Per Serving**:

- Protein Counts: 25 g

- Total Fats: 33 g

- Calories: 403

- Net Carbohydrates: 1.5 g

**Ingredients**:

- Ribeye steak (1 - 8 oz./226 g)

- Steakhouse seasoning (1 tbsp.)

- Wine vinegar (1 tsp.)

- Olive oil (1 tbsp.)

- Green salad mix (2 cups/150 g)

**Preparation Technique:**

1. Use the steak seasoning to prepare the steak and cook to your liking. Let it rest until cooled.

2. Arrange all of the salad fixings. Toss and drizzle with oil.

3. Slice the steak into bite-sized strips.

4.  Place the salad on two serving dishes and sprinkle the steak bits on top.

5.  Use your favorite dressing if desired - but count the carbs.

# Thai Pork Salad

**Servings**: 2

**Nutritional Facts Per Serving**:

- Protein Counts: 29 g

- Total Fats: 33 g

- Calories: 461

- Net Carbohydrates: 5.2 g

**Ingredients**:

*The Sauce:*

- Juice & zest of (1 lime)

- Chopped cilantro (2 tbsp.)

- Tomato paste (2 tbsp.)

- Soy sauce (2 tbsp. + 2 tsp.)

- Red curry paste (1 tsp.)

- Five Spice (1 tsp.)

- Fish sauce (1 tsp.)

- Red pepper flakes (.25 tsp.)

- Rice wine vinegar (1 tbsp. + 1 tsp.)

- Mango extract (.5 tsp.)

- Liquid stevia (10 drops)

*The Salad:*

- Romaine lettuce (2 cups/150 g)

- Pulled pork (10 oz./283 g)

- Medium chopped red bell pepper (¼ of 1)

- Chopped cilantro (.25 cup/15 grams)

## Preparation Technique:

1. Zest half of the lime and chop the cilantro. Mix all of the sauce fixings.

2. Blend the barbecue sauce components and set aside.

3. Pull the pork apart and make the salad. Pour glaze over the pork with a bit of the sauce.

# Vegetarian Club Salad

**Servings**: 3

**Nutritional Facts Per Serving**:

- Protein Counts: 17 g

- Total Fats: 26 g

- Calories: 330

- Net Carbohydrates: 5 g

**Ingredients**:

- Mayonnaise (2 tbsp.)

- Sour cream (2 tbsp.)

- Garlic powder (.5 tsp.)

- Dried parsley (1 tsp.)

- Onion powder (.5 tsp.)

- Milk (1 tbsp.)

- Dijon mustard (1 tbsp.)

- Large hard-boiled eggs (3)

- Cheddar cheese (4 oz./125 g)

- Cherry tomatoes (.5 cup/100 g)

- Diced cucumber (1 cup/140 g)

- Torn romaine lettuce (3 cups/225 g)

## Preparation Technique:

1. Slice the hard-boiled eggs and cube the cheese. Cut the tomatoes into halves and dice the cucumber. Place the containers to the side for now.

2. Prepare the dressing (dried herbs, mayo, and sour cream) mixing well.

3. Add one tablespoon of milk to the mixture - and another if it's too thick.

4. Layer the salad with the vegetables, cheese, and egg slices. Scoop a spoonful of mustard in the center along with a drizzle of dressing.

5. Toss well and serve.

6. *Notes:* The nutritional counts are based on two tablespoons of dressing.

# Asiago Tomato Soup

**Servings**: 4

**Nutritional Facts Per Serving**:

- Protein Counts: 9 g

- Total Fats: 26 g

- Calories: 302

- Net Carbohydrates: 8.75 g

**Ingredients**:

- Tomato paste (1 small can)

- Minced garlic (1 tsp.)

- Oregano (1 tsp.)

- Heavy whipping cream (1 cup/250 ml/8 fl. oz./226 g)

- Water (.25 cup/59 g)

- Pepper and salt (as desired)

- Asiago cheese (.75 cup/75 g)

**Preparation Technique**:

1. Pour the minced garlic and tomato paste in a Dutch oven and add the cream. Gently whisk.

2. As it begins to boil, blend in small amounts of cheese.

Pour in the water and simmer 4 to 5 minutes.

3.  Serve with pepper as desired.

# Beef & Carrot Soup - Instant Pot

**Servings**: 4

**Nutritional Facts Per Serving:**

- Protein Counts: 25 g

- Total Fats: 65 g

- Calories: 328

- Net Carbohydrates: 3 g

**Ingredients:**

- Beef stew meat (2 lb./900 g)

- Pepper & Salt (as desired)

- Cooking oil (2 tbsp.)

- Tomato paste (1 tbsp.)

- Garlic cloves (4)

- Sliced onion (1)

- Sliced carrots (4 peeled)

- Beef broth (3 cups/720 g)

- Bay leaves (2)

- Thyme sprigs (6)

- Water (1 cup/236 g)

**Preparation Technique:**

1. Dust the salt and pepper over the chopped beef.

2. Warm up the Instant Pot using the sauté function. Pour in the oil and add the beef. Sauté for 4 to 5 minutes until browned.

3. Stir in the onions, garlic, and carrots. Simmer 2 minutes and toss in the bay leaves, thyme, broth, and tomato paste. Stir well.

4. Secure the lid and set the timer for 30 minutes – manual setting.

5. When the set time is elapsed, natural release the pressure for 8-10 minutes and open the lid.

6. Season and enjoy warm.

# Beef Stew

**Servings**: 6

**Nutritional Facts Per Serving**:

- Protein Counts: 27 g

- Total Fats: 7 g

- Calories: 222

- Net Carbohydrates: 9 g

**Ingredients**:

- Beef broth (1 cup)

- Hot sauce (2 tsp.)

- Prepackaged chili mix (1 tbsp.)

- Stew beef (5 lb./2265 g)

- Worcestershire sauce (1 tbsp.)

- Chili-ready diced tomatoes (2 cans - 14.5 oz./410 g each)

- Salt (as desired)

**Preparation Technique:**

1. Use the high temperature setting on the slow cooker and toss in all of the fixings.

2. Prepare for six hours. The meat needs to be broken apart and cooked for an additional two hours. Add a pinch of salt. Serve when it's ready.

# Chicken Chowder - Crockpot

**Servings**: 4

**Nutritional Facts Per Serving**:

- Protein Counts: 40 g

- Total Fats: 28.8 g

- Calories: 457

- Net Carbohydrates: 7.5 g

**Ingredients**:

- Garlic clove (1)

- Cilantro (1 tbsp.)

- Small onion (1)

- Cream cheese (8 oz./225 g)

- Chicken broth (1 cup/240 g)

- Chicken breasts - skinless & boneless (1 lb./454 g)

- Diced tomatoes (14.5 oz./411 g)

- Diced jalapeno (.5 oz./15 g)

- Freshly squeezed lime juice (1.6 oz./45 g)

- Black pepper (1 tbsp.)

- Salt (1 tsp.)

**Preparation Technique:**

1. Chop the garlic and cilantro. Dice the onion and jalapeno.

2. Combine all of the fixings in the crockpot. Prepare on the low temperature setting for six to nine hours or high for four hours.

3. Once it is done, shred the chicken in the pot using two forks.

4. Serve or store in the fridge for later.

# Creamy Asparagus Soup

**Servings**: 2

**Nutritional Facts Per Serving**:

- Protein Counts: 7 g

- Total Fats: 13 g

- Calories: 157

- Net Carbohydrates: 3 g

**Ingredients**:

- Asparagus – save the juices (15 oz. can/425 g)

- Chicken broth (1.5 cups/362 g)

- Onion powder (.5 tsp.)

- Marjoram (.25 tsp.)

- Black pepper (.25 tsp.)

- Garlic powder (.25 tsp.)

- Heavy cream (.25 cup/57 g)

- Salt (as desired)

- Fresh parsley (1 tbsp.)

## Preparation Technique:

1.  Remove the asparagus from the can. Add enough broth to fill the asparagus can to make a full container.

2.  Roughly chop the asparagus and add the juices into a medium pot. Puree with an immersion blender until creamy. Stir in the seasonings and reduce the heat. Add the parsley and simmer until it's hot.

# Egg Drop Soup

**Servings**: 6

**Nutritional Facts Per Serving**:

- Protein Counts: 11 g
- Total Fats: 22 g
- Calories: 255
- Net Carbohydrates: 3 g

**Ingredients**:

- Vegetable broth (2 quarts/1900 ml)
- Freshly chopped ginger (1 tbsp.)
- Turmeric (1 tbsp.)
- Sliced chili pepper (1 small)
- Coconut aminos (2 tbsp.)
- Minced garlic cloves (2)
- Large eggs (4)
- Mushrooms (2 cups sliced/150 g)
- Chopped spinach (4 cups/900 g)
- Sliced spring onions (2 medium)
- Freshly chopped cilantro (2 tbsp.)

- Black pepper (to your liking)

- Pink Himalayan (1 tsp.)

- For serving: Olive oil (6 tbsp.)

## Preparation Technique:

1. Prep the Fixings: Grate the ginger root and turmeric. Mince the garlic cloves and slice the peppers and mushrooms.

2. Chop the chard stalks and leaves. Separate the stems from the leaves. Dump the vegetable stock into a soup pot and simmer until it begins to boil. Toss in the garlic, ginger, turmeric, chard stalks, mushrooms, coconut aminos, and chili peppers. Boil for approximately five minutes.

3. Fold in the chard leaves and simmer for one minute.

4. Whip the eggs in a dish and add them slowly to the soup mixture. Stir until the egg is done and set it on the counter.

5. Slice the onions and chop the cilantro. Toss them into the pot.

6. Pour into serving bowls and drizzle with some olive oil (1 tbsp. per serving).

7. Serve warm or chilled.

# Kale - Sausage & Mushroom Soup

**Servings**: 6

**Nutritional Facts Per Serving**:

- Protein Counts: 14 g

- Total Fats: 20 g

- Calories: 259

- Net Carbohydrates: 4 g

**Ingredients**:

- Fresh kale (6.5 oz./5 g)

- Mushrooms (6.5 oz./184 g)

- Chicken bone broth (29 oz./822 g)

- Sausage (1 lb./453 g)

- Garlic (2 cloves)

**Preparation Technique:**

1. Chop the kale into bite-sized pieces. Slice the mushrooms and mince the garlic.

2. Remove the casings and cook the sausage.

3.  Pour in the broth with two cans of water. Boil using the
    medium temperature setting.

4.  Toss in the rest of the fixings and simmer for one hour
    using the low-temperature setting.

# Mexican Chicken Soup - Slow-Cooked

**Servings**: 6

**Nutritional Facts Per Serving**:

- Protein Counts: 28 g

- Total Fats: 23 g

- Calories: 400

- Net Carbohydrates: 5 g

**Ingredients**:

- Chicken thighs (1.5 lb./680 g)

- Chicken broth (15 oz./425 g)

- Chunky salsa – ex. Tostitos (15.5 oz./439 g)

- Pepper Jack/Monterey cheese (8 oz./118 g)

**Preparation Technique:**

1. Cut out any bones and remove the fat from the chicken. Arrange them in the slow cooker.

2. Mix in the rest of the fixings. Prepare using the low setting (6-8 hrs.) or the high setting (3 to 4 hrs.).

3. When the time is up, remove and shred the chicken. Put it back in the cooker to mingle with the juices for a minute or so.

4.  Stir and serve - right out of the cooker.

# No-Beans Chili Delight

**Servings**: 6

**Nutritional Facts Per Serving**:

- Protein Counts: 26 g

- Total Fats: 14 g

- Calories: 263

- Net Carbohydrates: 5 g

**Ingredients**:

- Water (3 cups/710 g)

- Ground beef (1.5 lb./453 g)

- Cumin (.75 tsp.)

- Black pepper (.75 tsp.)

- Cinnamon (.25 tsp.)

- Minced garlic cloves (2)

- Chopped onion (.25 cup/25 g)

- Worcestershire sauce (1 tsp.)

- Bay leaves (3)

- Chili powder (2 tbsp.)

- Salt (1.5 tsp.)

- Allspice (.5 tsp.)

- Red pepper (.5 tsp.)

- Tomato paste (6 oz./170 g)

- Sliced black olives (2.25 oz./64 g)

- Finely chopped chili peppers (.25 cup/45 g)

**Preparation Technique:**

1. Break apart the ground beef in a large stew pot on the stovetop. Drain away the juices.

2. Combine with the rest of the fixings. Bring to a boil.

3. Simmer two hours and serve.

# Chapter 6: Poultry Options

## Asparagus - Stuffed Chicken

**Servings**: 4

**Nutritional Facts Per Serving**:

- Protein Counts: 32 g

- Total Fats: 25 g

- Calories: 377

- Net Carbohydrates: 2 g

**Ingredients**:

- Asparagus spears (12 or about .5 lb./226 g)

- Bacon pieces (8 slices)

- Chicken tenders (8 or about 1 lb./453 g)

- Salt (.5 tsp.)

- Black pepper (.25 tsp.)

**Preparation Technique:**

1. Set the oven temperature setting to reach 400F/204C.

2. Prepare a baking sheet and lay out two slices of bacon.

3. Season the chicken tenders with pepper and salt and

place them on top of the bacon.

4.  Add three spears of asparagus and wrap with the bacon and chicken to hold it all together.

5. Continue the process and bake for 40 minutes. The bacon should be crispy and the asparagus tender.

# Basil Stuffed Chicken Breasts

**Servings**: 2

**Nutritional Facts Per Serving**:

- Protein Counts: 41 g

- Total Fats: 25 g

- Calories: 405

- Net Carbohydrates: 1 g

**Ingredients**:

- Bone-in & skin-on breasts of chicken (2)

- Cream cheese (2 tbsp.)

- Shredded cheese (2 tbsp.)

- Garlic paste (.25 tsp.)

- Finely chopped basil leaves (3-4)

**Preparation Technique:**

1. Set the oven temperature at 375F/191C.

2. Prepare the stuffing using the fixings (cheese, cream cheese, basil, and garlic paste).

3. Peel the skin back on one side of the chicken and add half of the stuffing.

4.  Smooth it down and do the same to the other half.

5.  Roast it for 45 minutes or until it reaches 165F/75C (internal temperature).

# Cheesy Chicken Nuggets

**Servings**: 6

**Nutritional Facts Per Serving**:

- Protein Counts: 18 g

- Total Fats: 17 g

- Calories: 243

- Net Carbohydrates: 2 g

**Ingredients**:

- Egg (1)

- Cooked chicken (2 cups/ 250 g)

- Cream cheese (8 oz./225 g)

- Almond flour (.25 cup/24 g)

- Garlic salt (1 tsp.)

**Preparation Technique:**

1. Warm the oven to reach 350F/177C.

2. Lightly spritz a baking pan using a cooking oil spray or layer it with a sheet of parchment baking paper.

3. Shred the chicken using a food processor. Try using a combination of white and dark meat - your choice.

4.  Stir in the rest of the fixings and combine well.

5.  Drop the nugget mixture onto the prepared baking tin. Bake until firm and slightly browned (12 to 14 minutes).

# Chicken Mozzarella & Pesto Casserole

**Servings**: 6-8

**Nutritional Facts Per Serving**:

- Protein Counts: 38 g

- Total Fats: 30 g

- Calories: 451

- Net Carbohydrates: 3 g

**Ingredients**:

- Cooking oil (as needed)

- Grilled & cubed chicken breasts (2 lb./907 g)

- Unchilled cream cheese (8 oz./225 g)

- Cubed mozzarella (8 oz./225 g)

- Shredded mozzarella (8 oz./225 g)

- Pesto (.25 cup/62 g)

- Heavy cream (.5 cup/119 g as desired)

**Preparation Technique**:

1. Warm the oven to reach 400F/205C. Spritz a casserole dish using a cooking oil spray.

2. Combine the heavy cream, pesto, and softened cream

cheese.

3. Add the chicken and cubed mozzarella into the greased dish.

4. Bake it for 25 to 30 minutes.

5. *Cooking Tip*: Use 1/2 cup/96 g of cream if you prefer a thinner sauce or 1/4 cup/32 g for a thicker choice.

# Crack Chicken - Slow-Cooked

**Servings**: 4

**Nutritional Facts Per Serving**:

- Protein Counts: 55 g

- Total Fats: 45 g

- Calories: 647

- Net Carbohydrates: 1 g

**Ingredients**:

- Chicken breasts (4)

- Hidden Valley Original Ranch Seasoning (1 packet)

- Cream cheese (16 oz./450 g)

- Hot sauce (as desired)

**Preparation Technique:**

1. Chop the cheese into chunks.

2. Toss all of the fixings into the slow cooker.

3. Set the timer for six to eight hours using the low setting or four to six hours on the high cycle.

4. The internal temperature in the thickest part should reach 165F/74C.

5. Remove the chicken and shred it and mix with the fixings before serving.

# Creamy Onion Chicken

**Servings**: 4

**Nutritional Facts Per Serving**:

- Protein Counts: 38 g

- Total Fats: 26 g

- Calories: 400

- Net Carbohydrates: 3 g

**Ingredients**:

- Butter (2 tbsp. /28.3 g)

- Chicken breast halves (4 - no skin or bones)

- Whole green spring onion (1)

- Sour cream (8 oz./245 g)

- Sea salt (.5 tsp.)

## Preparation Technique:

1. Warm a frying pan to melt the butter using the med-high setting.

2. Lower the temperature setting to med-low and arrange the chicken in the pan. Cover the pan and cook the chicken for about ten minutes.

3. Chop the onion using the white and green sections. Flip

the chicken breasts. Place the lid back on the pan and simmer another eight to nine minutes or until it's done.

4. Toss in the onion and cook an additional one or two minutes.

5. Take it from the burner. Blend in the sour cream and salt.

6. Wait for about five minutes. Serve with your favorite veggies.

# Green Beans & Chicken

**Servings**: 3

**Nutritional Facts Per Serving**:

- Protein Counts: 19 g

- Total Fats: 11 g

- Calories: 196

- Net Carbohydrates: 4 g

**Ingredients**:

- Olive oil (2 tbsp.)

- Trimmed green beans (1 cup/150 g)

- Whole chicken breasts (2)

- Halved cherry tomatoes (8)

- Italian seasoning (1 tbsp.)

**Preparation Technique:**

1. Heat a skillet using the medium heat temperature setting. Pour in the oil.

2. Sprinkle the chicken with pepper, salt, and Italian seasoning.

3. Arrange them in the pan to cook for 10 minutes on each side.

4. Add the tomatoes and beans. Simmer another 5 to 7 minutes and serve

# Kung Pao Chicken

**Servings**: 4

**Nutritional Facts Per Serving**:

- Protein Counts: 23 g

- Total Fats: 18 g

- Calories: 264

- Net Carbohydrates: 4 g

**Ingredients**:

*The Chicken:*

- Coconut oil (1 tbsp.)

- Red bell pepper (⅓ of 1 medium)

- Celery (2 stalks)

- Peanuts (.25 cup/36 g)

- Ground ginger (1 tsp.)

- Minced garlic (.5 tsp.)

- Chicken thighs (4 skinless/boneless)

- *Optional:* Xanthan Gum (.25 tsp.)

*The Sauce:*

- Liquid aminos (.25 cup/79 g)

- Chicken broth (.25 cup/60 g)

- Chili garlic sauce/sriracha sauce (1.5 tbsp.)

- Sesame oil (1 tsp.)

- Rice wine vinegar (1 tsp.)

- Liquid stevia (30 drops)

**Preparation Technique:**

1. Heat a large skillet using the med-high temperature setting. Add the oil to heat.

2. Dice the pepper and celery into big chunks. Set them aside.

3. Chop the chicken into chunks and toss into the pan until done.

4. Meanwhile, make the sauce using all of the ingredients. Whisk it and set it aside.

5. Fold the prepared veggies into the pan with the chicken and simmer for two to three minutes. Add the peanuts and toast them for another few minutes.

6. Add the garlic and ginger to the mixture, stir, and mix in with the sauce. Stir in the xanthan gum as the sauce starts to thicken.

7. Serve with your favorite side like cauliflower rice.

# Lemon Chicken with Angel Hair Pasta

**Servings**: 3

**Nutritional Facts Per Serving**:

- Protein Counts: 39 g

- Total Fats: 16 g

- Calories: 325

- Net Carbohydrates: 2 g

**Ingredients**:

- Chicken breast (1 lb./454 g)

- Large lemon (1)

- Shirataki angel hair noodles (2, 7-oz./200 g pkg.)

- Garlic (1 large clove)

- XCT oil/another cooking oil (1 tbsp.)

- Organic garlic (1 large clove)

- Dried oregano (.5 tsp.) or Minced fresh oregano - leaves only (1 tsp.)

- Himalayan pink salt (.5 tsp.)

- Butter or ghee (2 tbsp.)

- Collagelatin/another grass-fed gelatin (1 tbsp.)

- Fresh oregano - leaves only (1-2 tbsp.)

**Preparation Technique:**

1. Squeeze the juice and zest from the lemon into separate containers.

2. Prepare the noodles, and rinse for 15 seconds. Boil for two minutes in a saucepan of boiling water. Drain the noodles and arrange them in a dry skillet using the medium temperature heat setting. "Dry roast" them for one minute. Cool them in the pan for two to three minutes.

3. Using the med-high temperature setting, warm a cast-iron skillet with oil.

4. Mince the chicken into small pieces and toss into the skillet with the minced garlic, salt, and dried oregano.

5. Sauté until thoroughly cooked for about eight to ten minutes. Stir occasionally. Transfer the chicken into a mixing bowl and set it aside.

6. Lower the pan temperature setting to medium. Pour in the lemon juice to deglaze the pan. Add butter and whisk in the gelatin to finish.

7. Mix the noodles and chicken back into the skillet, tossing thoroughly to combine.

8. Serve topped with lemon zest and a garnish of fresh oregano.

# Oven-Baked Pan-Fried Chicken

**Servings**: 4

**Nutritional Facts Per Serving**:

- Protein Counts: 48 g

- Total Fats: 19 g

- Calories: 392

- Net Carbohydrates: 4 g

**Ingredients**:

- Ranch Seasoning Mix (1 oz. pkg./28 g)

- Chicken breasts (4 boneless - skinless)

- Olive oil (2 tbsp.)

- Chicken broth (.75 cup/240 g)

- Unsalted butter (2 tbsp.)

**Preparation Technique:**

1. Set the oven at 425F/218C.

2. Season the chicken with two teaspoons of the Hidden Valley Seasoning.

3. Heat the oil in a large, oven-proof skillet using the med-high temperature setting.

4. Add and sauté the chicken until browned (5 min.). Flip
   it over and sauté for one more minute.

5. Pour in the chicken broth, butter, and remaining
   seasoning mix. Wait for it to boil, stirring gently to
   combine.

6. Transfer the whole pan into the preheated oven and
   roast until the chicken is cooked thoroughly (15 min.).
   Baste the chicken twice throughout the cooking cycle
   with the seasoned broth.

7. Serve warm with any remaining sauce on the side.

# Pizza Chicken Casserole

**Servings**: 6

**Nutritional Facts Per Serving**:

- Protein Counts: 35 g

- Total Fats: 24 g

- Calories: 383

- Net Carbohydrates: 4 g

**Ingredients**:

- Cooked chicken breast sliced or cubed (2 lb./900 g)

- Cream cheese (8 oz./225 g)

- Dried minced garlic (1 tsp.)

- Marinara sauce no sugar added (1 cup/225 g)

- Shredded mozzarella (8 oz./225 g)

- Also Needed: 9 by 13 baking dish

**Preparation Technique:**

1. Set the oven temperature at 350F/175C.

2. Slice or cube the chicken and toss it into the baking dish.

3. Mix the garlic and cream cheese in a bowl and drop by

the spoonful onto the chicken.

4. Dump the sauce over the top and add the shredded mozzarella.

5. Set the timer to bake for 30 minutes. It's ready when the cheese is bubbly and melted.

# Rosemary Ranch Chicken Kabobs

**Servings**: 6

**Nutritional Facts Per Serving**:

- Protein Counts: 32 g

- Total Fats: 16 g

- Calories: 284

- Net Carbohydrates: 1 g

**Ingredients**:

- Olive oil (.33 cup/72 g)

- Worcestershire sauce (2 tbsp.)

- Ranch seasoning (1.5 tbsp.)

- Lemon juice (2 tbsp.)

- Minced fresh rosemary (1 tbsp. + more for the garnish)

- Chicken breasts (4 boneless - skinless)

- Also Needed: Wooden skewers (8–10)

**Preparation Technique**:

1. Soak the skewers for about 20 minutes.

2. Whisk the rosemary, seasoning, lemon juice, Worcestershire sauce, and oil in a mixing bowl.

3. Cut the chicken into 1-inch cubes and add to the bowl. Marinate for about half an hour or overnight.

4. Warm the grill using the med-high setting. Grease the grates and thread the chicken onto the skewers. Discard the marinade.

5. Place the breasts on the grill for 10-12 minutes, rotating about halfway through the cycle.

6. Garnish with rosemary and serve it piping hot with our favorite veggies.

# Stuffed Chicken with Bacon & Asparagus

**Servings**: 4

**Nutritional Facts Per Serving**:

- Protein Counts: 32 g

- Total Fats: 25 g

- Calories: 377

- Net Carbohydrates: 2 g

**Ingredients**:

- Chicken tenders (9, 1 lb./453 g)

- Asparagus spears (12 or .5 lb./250 g)

- Black pepper (.25 tsp.)

- Salt (.5 tsp.)

- Bacon slices (8)

**Preparation Technique:**

1. Heat the oven in advance at 400F/205C.

2. Stretch the bacon on a baking tin and arrange two tenders over that.

3.  Add the asparagus, pepper, and salt. Fold and wrap the four bundles.

4.  Bake it for 40 minutes and serve.

# Chapter 7: Beef Options

## Bacon Burger Cabbage Stir Fry

**Servings**: 10

**Nutritional Facts Per Serving**:

- Protein Counts: 32 g

- Total Fats: 22 g

- Calories: 357

- Net Carbohydrates: 4.5 g

**Ingredients**:

- Ground beef (1 lb./455 g)

- Bacon (1 lb./455 g)

- Small onion (1)

- Minced cloves of garlic (3)

- Cabbage (1 lb./455 g or 1 small head)

**Preparation Technique:**

1. Dice the bacon and onion.

2. Combine the beef and bacon in a wok or large skillet. Prepare it until done and store it in a bowl to keep warm.

3. Mince the onion and garlic. Toss both into the hot grease.

4. Slice and toss in the cabbage and stir-fry until wilted.

5. Blend in the meat and combine. Sprinkle with pepper and salt as desired

# Barbacoa Beef – Instant Pot

**Servings**: 9

**Nutritional Facts Per Serving**:

- Protein Counts: 24 g

- Total Fats: 4.5 g

- Calories: 153

- Net Carbohydrates: 2 g

**Ingredients**:

- Eye round/bottom round roast (3 lb./1361 g)

- Black pepper (as desired)

- Kosher salt (2.5 tsp.)

- Water (1 cup/236 g)

- Medium onion (half of 1)

- Lime (1 juiced)

- Garlic cloves (5)

- Chipotles in adobo sauce (2-4 /to taste)

- Oregano (1 tbsp.)

- Ground cumin (1 tbsp.)

- Oil (1 tsp.)

- Bay leaves (3)

- Ground cloves (0.5 tsp.)

## Preparation Technique:

1. Program the Instant Pot using the sauté function.

2. Discard the fat from the beef and slice it into three-inch segments. Sprinkle with pepper and salt.

3. Puree the water, cloves, chipotles, oregano, lime juice, onion, garlic, and cumin in a blender.

4. Mix the oil and brown the meat for about five minutes. Add the sauce (from the blender) and the bay leaves.

5. Cook for 65 minutes (sauté mode with the top on) until it's easily shredded with two forks. Add water if needed to ensure it remains moist.

6. When ready, arrange on a serving platter, shred, and add it back to the pot. Save the juices for later and trash the bay leaves.

7. Measure out 1.5 cups of the reserved juices and mix with ½ of a teaspoon of cumin and salt.

8. Serve once it has warmed up, and the flavors have blended.

# Beef Pizza

**Servings**: 4

**Nutritional Facts Per Serving**:

- Protein Counts: 44 g

- Total Fats: 45 g

- Calories: 610

- Net Carbohydrates: 2 g

**Ingredients**:

- Eggs (2 large)

- Ground beef (20 oz./ 567 g pkg.)

- Pepperoni (28 slices)

- Shredded cheddar cheese (.5 cup/113 g)

- Pizza sauce (.5 cup/113 g)

- Mozzarella cheese (4 oz./113 g)

- Also Needed: 1 Cast-iron skillet

**Preparation Technique:**

1. Combine the eggs, beef, and seasonings. Pour the mixture into the skillet to form the crust. Bake until the meat is done or for about 15 minutes.

2.  Take it out and add the sauce, cheese, and toppings.

3.  Place the pizza in the oven for a few minutes until the
    cheese has melted. Remove and serve.

# Cabbage Skillet Tacos

**Servings**: 4

**Nutritional Facts Per Ser**:

- Protein Counts: 30 g

- Total Fats: 21 g

- Calories: 325

- Net Carbohydrates: 4 g

**Ingredients**:

- Ground beef (1 lb./454 g)

- Salsa - ex. Pace Organic (.5 cup/113 g)

- Shredded cabbage (2 cups/200 g)

- Chili powder (2 tsp.)

- Shredded cheese (.75 cup/96 g)

**Preparation Technique:**

1. Brown the beef and drain the fat. Pour in the salsa, cabbage, and seasoning.

2. Cover and lower the heat. Simmer for 10 to 12 minutes using the medium heat temperature setting.

3. When the cabbage has softened, remove it from the heat and mix in the cheese.

4. Top it off using your favorite toppings, such as green onions or sour cream, and serve.

# Cheesy Steak Pinwheels

**Servings**: 6

**Nutritional Facts Per Serving**:

- Protein Counts: 55 g

- Total Fats: 20g

- Calories: 414

- Net Carbohydrates: 2 g

**Ingredients**:

- Flank steak (2 lb./907 g)

- Mozzarella cheese (8 oz./226 g pkg.)

- Spinach (1 bunch - 1.75 cups/224 g approximately)

**Preparation Technique:**

1. Warm the oven to reach 350F/175C.

2. Slice the steak into six portions and remove all of the 'hard' fat. Beat until thin with a mallet.

3. Shred the cheese using a food processor and sprinkle the steak. Roll it up and tie with a piece of cooking twine or a skewer.

4. Line the pan with the pinwheels and place it on a layer of spinach. Bake until done (25 minutes).

# Enchilada Skillet Dinner

**Servings**: 4

**Nutritional Facts Per Serving**:

- Protein Counts: 36 g

- Total Fats: 30 g

- Calories: 455

- Net Carbohydrates: 7 g

**Ingredients**:

- Small yellow onion (1)

- Ground beef (1.5 lb./680 g)

- Red enchilada sauce (1/3 cup/79 g)

- Chopped green onions (8)

- Diced Roma tomatoes (2)

- Shredded cheddar cheese (4 oz./125 g)

- Optional: Fresh cilantro

**Preparation Technique**:

1. Use a wok/skillet and sauté the yellow onion and beef. Drain the juices and add the green onions, tomato, and enchilada sauce.

2. Once it starts to boil, simmer for about five minutes. Sprinkle with the salt and cheese. Continue cooking until the cheese has melted.

3. Chop and stir in the cilantro. Serve over chopped lettuce and portion of sour cream (add the carbs).

# Feta-Stuffed Burgers

**Servings**: 2

**Nutritional Facts Per Serving**:

- Protein Counts: 41 g

- Total Fats: 48 g

- Calories: 607

- Net Carbohydrates: 1 g

**Ingredients**:

- Scallion (1)

- Ground beef & lamb (12 oz. total/340 g)

- Chopped mint leaves (2 tbsp.)

- Ghee (1 tbsp.)

- Dijon mustard (1 tbsp.)

- Crumbled feta cheese (2 oz./56 g)

- Pink salt and Black pepper (to your liking)

**Preparation Technique**:

1. Thinly slice the green and white parts of the scallion. Also, finely chop the fresh mint leaves. Crumble the feta.

2.  Combine the mustard with the mint and scallions. Stir in the beef and lamb. Mix well and shape into four patties. Sprinkle with salt and pepper.

3.  Press the feta cubes into two of the patties and place a patty on top (cheese in the middle). Seal it closed.

4.  Using the medium heat setting, melt the ghee and add the patties once the pan is hot. Cook each side for 5 minutes and serve.

# Ground Beef Keto Meatballs

**Servings**: 8-10

**Nutritional Facts Per Serving**:

- Protein Counts: 12.2 g

- Total Fats: 10.9 g

- Calories: 153

- Net Carbohydrates: 0.7 g

**Ingredients**:

- Large egg (1)

- Grated parmesan (.5 cup/50 g)

- Shredded mozzarella (.5 cup/50 g)

- Ground beef (1 lb./455 g)

- Minced garlic (1 tbsp.)

**Preparation Technique:**

1. Warm the oven to reach 400F/204C. Cover a baking tin with a sheet of parchment baking paper.

2. Combine all of the fixings using your hands.

3. Shape them into the desired sized meatballs.

4. Bake for 18-20 minutes. Cool slightly and serve.

# Meatloaf

**Servings**:

**Nutritional Facts Per Serving**:

- Protein Counts: 25 g

- Total Fats: 31 g

- Calories: 406

- Net Carbohydrates: 3 g

**Ingredients**:

- Ground beef (2 lb./907 g)

- Almond flour (.75 cup/72 g)

- Large eggs (2)

- Parmesan cheese (.5 cup/50 g)

- Original Ranch® Seasoning (1 packet)

- Optional: Unsweetened ketchup (.25 cup/60 g)

- Also Needed: 9x5-inch loaf pan

**Preparation Technique**:

1. Set the oven to reach 350F/177C. Grease the pan and set it aside.

2. Combine all of the fixings except the ketchup until it's

well blended but not overmixed.

3. Transfer the mixture into the loaf pan. Set a timer to bake it for 40 minutes. Transfer the pan from the oven and spread the top using the ketchup.

4.  Return the meatloaf into the oven and bake for another 20 minutes, until it's done (internal temperature reaches 160F/71C). If you don't use ketchup, bake for 60 minutes total.

5. Wait for at least 10 minutes before slicing.

# Monterey Mug Melt

**Servings**: 1

**Nutritional Facts Per Serving**:

- Protein Counts: 22 g

- Total Fats: 18 g

- Calories: 268

- Net Carbohydrates: 4 g

**Ingredients**:

- Roast beef deli slices (2 oz./57 g)

- Diced green chilis (1.5 tbsp.)

- Sour cream (1 tbsp.)

- Shredded pepper jack cheese (1.5 oz./42 g)

**Preparation Technique:**

1. Tear the roast beef apart and layer it in the bottom of the dish.

2. Spread about ½ of a tablespoon of the sour cream and ½ tablespoon of the green chili. Layer ½ ounce of the pepper cheese. Follow with another layer.

3. Microwave for one to two minutes until the cheese melts and serve.

# Skillet Steak - Nacho Style

**Servings**: 5

**Nutritional Facts Per Serving**:

- Protein Counts: 19 g

- Total Fats: 31 g

- Calories: 385

- Net Carbohydrates: 6 g

**Ingredients**:

- Cauliflower (1.5 lb./680 g)

- Turmeric (.5 tsp.)

- Chili powder (1 tsp.)

- Butter (1 tbsp.)

- Beef round tip steak (8 oz./226 g)

- Melted refined coconut oil (.33 cup/72 g)

- Shredded cheddar cheese (1 oz./28 g)

- Shredded Monterey Jack cheese (1 oz./28 g)

  *Optional Garnishes:*

- Sour cream (.33 cup/75 g)

- Canned - jalapeno slices (1 oz./28 g)

- Avocado (approx. 5 oz./93 g)

**Preparation Technique:**

1. Set the oven temperature setting at 400F/205C.

2. Prepare the cauliflower into chip-like shapes.

3. Combine the turmeric, chili powder, and coconut oil in a mixing dish.

4. Toss in the cauliflower and add it to a baking tin. Set the baking timer for 20 to 25 minutes.

5. Over med-high heat in a cast iron skillet, add the butter. Cook until both sides of the meat are done, flipping just once. Let it rest for 5-10 minutes. Thinly slice and sprinkle with some pepper and salt.

6. When done, transfer the florets to the skillet and add the steak strips. Top it off with the cheese and bake for 5-10 more minutes.

7. Serve with your favorite garnish.

8. Count the carbs for the added garnishes.

# Slow-Cooked London Broil

**Servings**: 4

**Nutritional Facts Per Serving**:

- Protein Counts: 47 g

- Total Fats: 18 g

- Calories: 409

- Net Carbohydrates: 2.5 g

**Ingredients**:

- London broil (2 lb./907 g)

- Dijon mustard (1 tbsp.)

- Reduced sugar ketchup (2 tbsp.)

- Minced garlic (2 tsp.)

- Coconut Aminos/ your choice soy sauce substitute (2 tbsp.)

- Coffee (.5 cup/68 g)

- Chicken broth (.5 cup/120 g)

- White wine (.25 cup/120 g)

- Onion powder (2 tsp.)

**Preparation Technique:**

1.  Place the beef in the cooker. Cover both sides with the mustard, soy sauce, ketchup, and minced garlic.

2.  Pour the liquid ingredients into the cooker and give it a sprinkle of the onion powder.

3.  Cook for four to six hours.

4.  When the timer buzzes, shred the meat. Combine with the juices and serve.

# Spinach-Mozzarella Stuffed Burgers

**Servings**: 4

**Nutritional Facts Per Serving**:

- Protein Counts: 36 g

- Total Fats: 29 g

- Calories: 414

- Net Carbohydrates: 1 g

**Ingredients**:

- Ground chuck (1.5 lb./680 g)

- Salt (1 tsp.)

- Black pepper (.75 tsp.)

- Firmly packed fresh spinach (2 cups/450 g)

- Grated parmesan cheese (2 tbsp.)

- Shredded mozzarella cheese (.5 cup/64 g or 4 oz.)

**Preparation Technique:**

1. Mix the ground beef, pepper, and salt.

2. Scoop about one-third of a cup of the mixture and shape into eight patties (½-inch thickness). Pop them into the fridge.

3. Prepare a pan of water and add the spinach using the med-high temperature setting. Place a lid on the pan and cook until it's wilted (2 min.). Drain and let it cool. Chop the spinach and toss it into a bowl with parmesan and mozzarella cheese.

4. Scoop about one-quarter of a cup of the stuffing and mound it into the center of four patties. Cover with the remaining four patties and seal the edges by pressing firmly together.

5. Press on the top to flatten slightly into a single thick patty.

6. Warm a grill using the med-high setting.

7. Grill the burgers for five to six minutes per side and garnish as desired before serving.

# Stroganoff

**Servings**: 1

**Nutritional Facts Per Serving**:

- Protein Counts: 39 g

- Total Fats: 28 g

- Calories: 447

- Net Carbohydrates: 6 g

**Ingredients**:

- Lean ground beef (1 lb./455 g)

- Sliced mushrooms (8 oz./124 g)

- Minced cloves of garlic (2)

- Butter (2 tbsp.)

- Sour cream (1.25 cups/287 g)

- Water or dry white wine (.33 cup/78 g)

- Lemon juice (1 tsp.)

- Dried parsley (1 tsp.)

- Paprika (.25 tsp.)

- Optional: Freshly chopped parsley (1 tbsp.)

**Preparation Technique:**

1. Slice/dice the mushrooms and garlic. Heat a skillet and melt one tablespoon of butter. Sauté the garlic and mushrooms, adding the beef, salt, and pepper.

2. Add the remainder of the butter, mushrooms, and the wine/water to the pan. Cook until half of the liquid is reduced, and the mushrooms are soft.

3. Take them away from the heat and add the paprika and sour cream.

4. Using low heat, stir in the meat, and lemon juice. Use additional spices for flavoring if desired.

# Chapter 8: Pork & Lamb Options

## Bacon & Brussels Sprouts

**Servings**: 6

**Nutritional Facts Per Serving**:

- Protein Counts: 7.9 g

- Total Fats: 6.9 g

- Calories: 113

- Net Carbohydrates: 3.9 g

**Ingredients**:

- Brussels sprouts (16 oz./176 g)

- Bacon (16 oz./453 g)

- Black pepper (as desired)

**Preparation Technique:**

1.  Warm the oven to reach 400F/204C.

2.  Prepare a baking tray with a layer of parchment baking paper.

3.  Use sheers or a sharp knife to slice the bacon into small lengthwise pieces.

4.  Add the sprouts and bacon to the prepared ban with a

shake of pepper.

5.  Bake it for dinner and set a timer for 35 to 40 minutes until the bacon is crunchy and sprouts are lightly browned.

# Jamaican Jerk Pork Roast

**Servings**: 12

**Nutritional Facts Per Serving**:

- Protein Counts: 23 g

- Total Fats: 20 g

- Calories: 282

- Net Carbohydrates: 0 g

**Ingredients**:

- Olive oil (1 tbsp.)

- Pork shoulder (4 lb./1814 g)

- Broth or beef stock (.5 cup/120 g)

- Jamaican Jerk spice blend (.25 cup/60 g)

- Also Needed: Dutch oven/regular oven

**Preparation Technique:**

1. Rub the roast well the oil and coat with the jerk spice blend.

2. Use the Dutch oven to sear the roast on all sides. Add the beef broth.

3. Cover the pot and simmer for about four hours using the low heat setting. (You can also bake it for 3 hours at 375F/191C.)

4. Shred and serve.

# Kalua Pork & Cabbage

**Servings**: 12

**Nutritional Facts Per Serving**:

- Protein Counts: 22 g

- Total Fats: 13 g

- Calories: 227

- Net Carbohydrates: 4 g

**Ingredients**:

- Boneless pork shoulder butt (3 lb./1360 g)

- Head of cabbage (1 medium - approx. 2 lb./907 g)

- Bacon (7 strips - divided)

- Coarse sea salt (1 tbsp.)

- Suggested: 6-quart slow cooker

**Preparation Technique:**

1. Coarsely chop the cabbage. Trim the fat from the roast.

2. Layer most of the bacon in the cooker. Dust the salt over the roast and add to the slow cooker on top of the bacon. Place the rest of the bacon on top.

3. Close the top and cook on low for eight to ten hours.

4.  At that time, drop in the cabbage, and cook covered for another hour until the cabbage is tender. (Times may vary depending on the size of the cooker.)

5.  When the roast is done, remove it and shred. Arrange the cabbage in the serving dish using a slotted spoon to remove the juices.

6.  Use some of the slow cooker juices on the side for dipping.

# Pork Kabobs

**Servings**: 4

**Nutritional Facts Per Serving**:

- Protein Counts: 33.7 g

- Total Fats: 8.6 g

- Net Carbohydrates: 3.3 g

**Ingredients**:

- Hot sauce (2 tsp.)

- Sunflower seed butter (3 tbsp.)

- Minced garlic (1 tbsp.)

- Keto-friendly soy sauce (1 tbsp.)

- Water (1 tbsp.)

- Medium green pepper (1)

- Crushed red pepper (.5 tsp.)

- Squared pork for kebabs (1 lb./454 g)

**Preparation Technique:**

1. Warm the oven or grill using the broil or the high heat setting.

2. In a processor or blender, combine the water with the

red pepper, soy sauce, garlic, butter, and hot sauce.

3. Slice the pork into squares. Cover with the marinade and rest for 1 hour.

4. Chop the peppers to fit the skewer. Thread the skewers alternating the pork and peppers.

5. Broil using the high temperature setting for five minutes per side.

# Stuffed Pork Chops

**Servings**: 4

**Nutritional Facts Per Serving**:

- Protein Counts: 102 g

- Total Fats: 38 g

- Calories: 778

- Net Carbohydrates: 1 g

**Ingredients**:

- Bacon (3 slices)

- Thick-cut pork chops (4)

- Feta cheese (3 oz./85 g)

- Cream cheese (2 oz./60 g)

- Blue cheese (3 oz./85 g)

- Green onion (.33 cup/50 g)

- Garlic powder (1 pinch)

- Black pepper and salt (to taste)

**Preparation Technique:**

1. Set the oven temperature to reach 350F/175C. Lightly grease a baking tin.

2. Prepare the bacon, reserving the grease, and set it aside for now.

3. Thoroughly mix the feta and blue cheese with the onions, bacon, and cream cheese.

4. Split the non-fat side of the pork and add the cheese mixture, garlic powder, salt, and pepper – closing with a toothpick or skewer. Sprinkle using the salt, pepper, and garlic powder.

5. Sear them using the bacon grease in the skillet for 1.5 minutes per side.

6. Arrange the chops on the baking pan and cook for 55 minutes. Wait for the chops rest for about three minutes.

# Quick & Easy Lamb Chops

**Servings**: 6

**Nutritional Facts Per Serving**:

- Protein Counts: 14 g

- Total Fats: 21 g

- Calories: 252

- Net Carbohydrates: 1 g

**Ingredients**:

- Lamb chops (6 - 4 oz. each/115 g each)

- Whole garlic cloves (4)

- Thyme sprigs (2)

- Ground thyme (1 tsp.)

- Olive oil (3 tbsp.)

- Black Pepper and Salt (1 tsp. each)

**Preparation Technique:**

1. Heat a skillet using the medium temperature setting. Once it's hot, add the olive oil.

2. Season the chops with the spices (pepper, thyme, and salt).

3. Arrange the chops in the skillet along with the garlic
   and sprigs of thyme.

4. Sauté about 3 to 4 minutes on each side and serve.

# Chapter 9: Healthy Dessert Options

## Almond Coconut Bars - Instant Pot

**Servings**: 8

**Nutritional Facts Per Serving**:

- Protein Counts: 5 g

- Total Fats: 25 g

- Calories: 253

- Net Carbohydrates: 2 g

**Ingredients**:

- Coconut oil (.5 cup/104 g)

- Almond flour (1.25 cups/120 g)

- Coconut flour (.25 cup/30 g)

- Eggs (2)

- Sugar substitute (3 tbsp.)

- Almond butter (2 tbsp.)

- Salt (.25 tsp.)

- Water (1 cup/236 g)

- Vanilla extract (1 tsp.)

## Preparation Technique:

1. Line the pan that fits in the cooker with the baking paper.

2. Combine all of the fixings in the food processor and add it to the pan.

3. Empty the water into the Instant Pot with the steamer rack. Arrange the pan in the cooker and secure the lid.

4. Set the timer for 15 minutes.

5. Naturally release the pressure and chill the pan until its room temperature.

6. Slice into six bars.

# Almond Pumpkin Seed Bars

**Servings**: 8

**Nutritional Facts Per Serving**:

- Protein Counts: 4.7 g

- Total Fats: 25 g

- Calories: 261.5

- Net Carbohydrates: 3.8 g

**Ingredients**:

- Almond flour (1 cup/96 g)

- Melted butter – divided (.25 cup/57 g)

- Erythritol – divided (.25 cup/57 g)

- Salt (.5 tsp.)

- Heavy cream (.25 cup/60 ml or 4 tbsp.)

- Cinnamon (.5 tsp.)

- Maple extract (1 tsp.)

- Xanthan gum (.25 tsp.)

- Toasted pumpkin seeds (.5 cup/59 g)

- Also Needed: 8 by 8-inch baking pan

"""

## Preparation Technique:

1. Set the oven at 400F/204C. Prepare a baking pan with a layer of parchment baking paper.

2. Combine 1/4 cup/ 32 g of the butter, almond flour, salt, and one tablespoon of the erythritol. Mix well.

3. Press the crust into the baking pan or dish. Bake it for 12 to 15 minutes and transfer to the countertop and let it cool.

4. Use a blender to combine the almond butter, the rest of the melted butter, xanthan gum, maple extract, cinnamon, and heavy cream. Blend until smooth and creamy. Scoop it into the prepared crust and top with the toasted pumpkin seeds.

5. Store in the fridge for a minimum of two hours; overnight is best.

6. Slice into eight squares.

# Amaretti Cookies

**Servings**: 16

**Nutritional Facts Per Serving**:

- Protein Counts: 2.5 g

- Total Fats: 8 g

- Calories: 86

- Net Carbohydrates: 1 g

**Ingredients**:

- Coconut flour (2 tbsp.)

- Cinnamon (.25 tsp.)

- Salt (.5 tsp.)

- Erythritol (.5 cup/181 g)

- Baking powder (.5 tsp.)

- Almond flour (1 cup/128 g)

- Eggs (2)

- Almond extract (.5 tsp.)

- Vanilla extract (.5 tsp.)

- Coconut oil (4 tbsp.)

- Sugar-free jam (2 tbsp.)

- Shredded coconut (1 tbsp.)

## Preparation Technique:

1. Cover the tin with a sheet of paper.

2. Warm up the oven to reach 400F/204C.

3. Sift the flour and combine all of the dry fixings.

4. After combined, work into the wet ones. Shape into 16 cookies.

5. Make a dent in the center of each one. Bake it for 15 to 17 minutes.

6. It is essential for them to cool a few minutes.

7. Add a dab of jam to each one and a sprinkle of the coconut bits.

# Blueberry Cupcakes

**Servings**: 12

**Nutritional Facts Per Serving**:

- Protein Counts: 4.4 g

- Total Fats: 11.4 g

- Calories: 138

- Net Carbohydrates: 2.8 g

**Ingredients**:

- Melted butter (1 stick)

- Granulated sweetener of choice (4 tbsp. or more to taste)

- Coconut flour (.5 cup/56 g)

- Baking powder (1 tsp.)

- Lemon juice (2 tbsp.)

- Vanilla (1 tsp.)

- Lemon zest (2 tbsp.)

- Eggs (8 medium)

- Fresh blueberries (1 cup/128 g)

## Preparation Technique:

1. Mix the melted butter, sweetener, coconut flour, baking powder, vanilla, lemon juice, and zest.

2. Add the eggs, one at a time. Mix well as you prepare the batter.

3. Taste the cupcake batter to ensure you have used enough sweetener and flavors to mask the subtle taste of coconut from the coconut flour.

4. Portion the batter into the tins.

5. Press in a few fresh blueberries in the batter of each cupcake.

6. Bake at 350F/177C for 15 minutes, or until golden on the outside, and cooked in the center.

7. Cover with sugar-free cream cheese frosting. Vanilla or lemon flavor is perfect. Garnish with fresh blueberries and lemon zest.

8. Icing/frosting is additional and optional.

# Chocolate Mini Cakes - Instant Pot

**Servings**: 2

**Nutritional Facts Per Serving**:

- Protein Counts: 15 g

- Total Fats: 12 g

- Calories: 193

- Net Carbohydrates: 9 g

**Ingredients**:

- Large eggs (2)

- Splenda/your favorite sweetener (2 tbsp.)

- Baking cocoa (.25 cup/30 g)

- Heavy cream (2 tbsp.)

- Baking powder (.5 tsp.)

- Vanilla extract (1 tsp.)

- Water (1 cup/236 g)

**Preparation Technique:**

1. Add the water and trivet into the Instant Pot.

2. Mix each of the dry fixings in one container.

3. In another dish, blend in the rest of the ingredients (eggs, cream, vanilla extract).

4. Spray the ramekins and fill each one halfway. Carefully add them to the cooker and secure the lid.

5. Prepare for nine minutes using the high-pressure setting.

6. Quick release the pressure and add to a plate to cool.

7. Cool before adding toppings or serve hot right out of the ramekin.

# Chocolate Mousse

**Servings**: 2

**Nutritional Facts Per Serving**:

- Protein Counts: 4 g

- Total Fats: 50 g

- Calories: 460

- Net Carbohydrates: 4 g

**Ingredients**:

- Butter (4 tbsp.)

- Cream cheese (4 tbsp.)

- Heavy whipping cream (1.5 tbsp.)

- Swerve or another natural sweetener (1 tbsp.)

- Unsweetened cocoa powder (1 tbsp.)

**Preparation Technique:**

1. Remove the butter and cream cheese from the fridge for about 30 minutes before time to prepare to become room temperature.

2. Chill a bowl and whisk the cream. Place back in the refrigerator for now.

3. Use a hand mixer to combine the sweetener, cream

cheese, cocoa powder, and butter until well mixed.

4.  Remove the refrigerated cream and fold it into the chocolate mixture using a rubber scraper.

5.  Portion it into two dessert bowls and chill for one hour.

# Easy Brownie Inug

**Servings**: 1

**Nutritional Facts Per Serving**:

- Protein Counts: 35 g

- Total Fats: 15 g

- Calories: 310

- Net Carbohydrates: 5 g

**Ingredients**:

- Granulated sweetener (1 tbsp.)

- Eggs (2)

- Heavy cream (1 tbsp.)

- Protein powder (1 scoop)

**Preparation Technique:**

1. Add the eggs, cream sweetener, and protein powder into the chosen mug. Mix well.

2. Place the cup in the microwave for one minute. Remove with caution and serve.

# No-Bake Coconut Cashew Protein Bars

**Servings**: 12

**Nutritional Facts Per Serving**:

- Protein Counts: 11 g

- Total Fats: 16 g

- Calories: 212

- Net Carbohydrates: 8.3 g

**Ingredients**:

- Coconut butter (.5 cup/109 g)

- Cashew butter (.25 cup/65 g)

- Coconut oil (.25 cup/33 g)

- Ground flaxseed (.66 cup/111 g)

- Protein powder –your favorite (1.33 cups/160 g)

- Coconut or cashew milk (.25 cup/60 g)

- Liquid stevia coconut drops (.5 tsp.)

- Optional Topping: Unsweetened coconut flakes

- Also Needed: 8 x 8-inch baking dish

**Preparation Technique:**

1. Soften the coconut butter, cashew butter, and coconut oil in the microwave or saucepan. Stir to incorporate and set aside to cool.

2. In another container, whisk the flaxseed and protein powder. Stir in the milk.

3. Taste test the cashew/coconut mixture for sweetness and adjust accordingly. Combine the rest of the fixings, mixing well.

4. Portion into 12 servings.

# Peanut Butter Protein Bars

**Servings**: 12

**Nutritional Facts Per Serving**:

- Protein Counts: 7 g

- Total Fats: 14 g

- Calories: 172

- Net Carbohydrates: 3 g

**Ingredients**:

- Coconut or olive oil – for the pan

- Almond meal (1.5 cups/141 g)

- Chunky peanut butter – keto-friendly (1 cup/250 g)

- Egg whites (2)

- Almonds (.5 cup/70 g)

- Cashews (.5 cup/75 g)

- Also Needed: Baking pan

**Preparation Technique**:

1. Set the oven at 350F/177C. Spritz a baking dish lightly with coconut or olive oil.

2. Combine all of the fixings and add them to the

prepared dish.

3. Bake 15 minutes and cut into 12 pieces once they're
   cooled.

4. Store in the fridge to keep them fresh.

# Pumpkin Bread

**Servings**: 8

**Nutritional Facts Per Serving**:

- Protein Counts: 8 g

- Total Fats: 26 g

- Calories: 311

- Net Carbohydrates: 5 g

**Ingredients**:

- Almond flour (1 cup/96 g)

- Libby's Canned Pumpkin (1 small can)

- Baking powder (.5 tsp.)

- Coconut flour (.5 cup/61 g)

- Heavy cream (.5 cup/170 g)

- Stevia (.5 cup/12 packets)

- Melted butter (1 stick)

- Eggs (4 large)

- Vanilla (1.5 tsp.)

- Pumpkin spice (2 tsp.)

**Preparation Technique:**

1.  Set the oven at 350F/177C.

2.  Grease a pan with a misting of coconut oil.

3.  Combine all of the fixings in a mixing container until light and fluffy.

4.  Empty the mixture into the chosen pan.

5.  Bake the bread for approximately 70 to 90 minutes.

# Pumpkin Cheesecake with Almond Pecan Crust

**Servings**: 16

**Nutritional Facts Per Serving**:

- Protein Counts: 8.6 g

- Total Fats: 20.5 g

- Calories: 245

- Net Carbohydrates: 5.9 g

**Ingredients**:

*The Crust:*

- Almonds (1 cup/85 g)

- Pecans (1 cup/125 g)

- Granular sucralose sweetener (2 -1 g packets)

- Butter - melted(3 tbsp.)

*The Filling:*

- Unchilled low-fat cream cheese (3 - 8 oz./227 g pkg.)

- Granular sucralose sweetener (.66 cup/133 g)

- Pumpkin puree (15 oz. can/425 g)

- Vanilla extract (1 tsp.)

- Ground ginger (.5 tsp.)

- Cinnamon (1 tsp.)

- Ground cloves (.25 tsp.)

- Salt (.25 tsp.)

- Eggs (3)

- Also Needed: 9-inch springform pan

**Preparation Technique:**

1. Warm the oven to reach 350F/177C.

2. Pulse the almonds and pecans in a food processor until ground - not pasty. Toss in the sweetener and butter; pulsing to combine. Press the crust into a pan and bake it about ten minutes until browned. Cool it for ten minutes.

3. Blend the cream cheese and 2/3 cup/85 g sweetener with an electric mixer until smooth or 2 to 3 minutes.

4. Mix in the vanilla extract, pumpkin, ginger, cinnamon, cloves, and salt until smooth (2 min.) Add in the eggs one at a time, mixing thoroughly after adding each one. Pour the batter into the crust.

5. Bake until it's just set in the center or when the filling jiggles but does not run (45 to 50 min.). Let it cool completely or about 30 minutes. Run a knife around the edge of the cheesecake, cover, and refrigerate it for a minimum of four hours before serving.

# Raspberry Coke – Slow Cooker

**Servings**: 10

**Nutritional Facts Per Serving**:

- Protein Counts: 10.4 g

- Total Fats: 32 g

- Calories: 362

- Net Carbohydrates: 6.7 g

**Ingredients**:

- Unsweetened shredded coconut (1 cup/100 g)

- Almond flour (2 cups/192 g)

- Swerve sweetener (.75- 1 cup/155 - 200 g)

- Large eggs (4)

- Powdered egg whites (.25 cup/21 g)

- Salt (.25 tsp.)

- Baking soda (2 tsp.)

- Melted coconut oil (.5 cup/104 g)

- Raspberries – fresh or frozen (1 cup/125 g)

- Coconut extract (1 tsp.)

- Almond or coconut milk (.75 cup/169 g)

- Sugar-free dark chocolate chips (.33 cup/50 g)

- Coconut oil or favorite cooking spray

- Recommended: 6-quart size

## Preparation Technique:

1. Spritz the inside of the slow cooker with some cooking oil spray.

2. Whisk the flour, sweetener, coconut, salt, baking soda, and powdered egg whites in a large mixing container.

3. Add the coconut or almond milk, eggs, coconut extract, and melted coconut oil. Stir well and fold in the chips and berries.

4. Spread the prepared batter into the cooker and cook on the low setting for three hours. Turn the unit off and let it cool.

5. Top with whipped cream and serve.

# Raspberry Fudge

**Servings**: 12

**Nutritional Facts Per Serving**:

- Protein Counts: 2.6 g

- Total Fats: 25.3 g

- Calories: 242

- Net Carbohydrates: 4.4 g

**Ingredients**:

- Cream cheese (16 oz./450 g)

- Butter (1 cup/227 g)

- White sugar substitute (.25 cup/50 g)

- Unsweetened cocoa powder (6 tbsp.)

- Heavy cream (2 tbsp.)

- Raspberry extract (1 tsp.)

- Vanilla extract (2 tsp.)

- Chopped walnuts (.33 cup/40 g)

**Preparation Technique:**

1. Take the cream cheese and butter out of the fridge ahead of time until it reaches room temperature.

2. Mix the cream cheese and butter in the mixing bowl with the mixer.

3. When smooth, mix with the rest of the fixings until well incorporated.

4. Microwave it using the high setting for 30 seconds. Blend with the mixer again until smooth.

5. Empty into the prepared pan (1-inch layer). Cover and chill for at least 2 hours in the fridge.

6. Slice into 12 portions.

7. Serve and enjoy or store for a delicious treat later.

8. Store in the refrigerator for the best results.

# Strawberry & Cream Cakes

**Servings**: 5

**Nutritional Facts Per Serving**:

- Protein Counts: 6 g

- Total Fats: 30 g

- Calories: 275

- Net Carbohydrates: 3.9 g

**Ingredients**:

- Eggs (3)

- Cream cheese (3 oz./6 tbsp.)

- Baking powder (.25 tsp.)

- Vanilla extract (.5 tsp.)

- Erythritol (2 tbsp.)

  *The Filling:*

- Strawberries (10)

- Heavy cream (1 cup/240 g)

**Preparation Technique**:

1. Cover a baking sheet with parchment paper. Warm the oven to reach 300 F/149C.

2.  Break the eggs and which just the egg *whites*. Whisk to form stiff peaks.

3.  In another dish, combine the cream cheese, egg *yolks*, vanilla extract, baking powder, and erythritol.

4.  Slowly add the egg mixtures together. Shape into cake forms and place them on the lined baking tin.

5.  Whip the heavy cream until thickened.

6.  Bake for 25-30 minutes. Let them cool and add the berries and cream.

# Smoothies

## Almond Lover Smoothie

**Servings**: 16 oz. glass

**Nutritional Facts Per Serving**:

- Protein Counts: 12 g

- Total Fats: 23 g

- Calories: 511

- Net Carbohydrates: 0 g

**Ingredients**:

- Medium banana (1)

- Almond milk (8 oz./1 cup/262 g)

- Plain non-fat Greek yogurt (.33 cup/94 g)

- Cooked oats (.33 cup/9 g)

- Almond butter (2 tbsp.)

- Almonds (5)

**Preparation Technique:**

1. Measure all of the fixings into the cup of your blender or favorite high-speed machine.

2. Pour the milk up to the max fill line. Blend until it is
   smooth and creamy.

# Blueberry - Banana Bread Smoothie

**Servings**: 2

**Nutritional Facts Per Serving**:

- Protein Counts: 3.1 g

- Total Fats: 23.3 g

- Calories: 270

- Net Carbohydrates: 4.7 g

**Ingredients**:

- Chia seeds (1 tbsp.)

- Golden flaxseed meal (3 tbsp.)

- Vanilla unsweetened coconut milk (2 cups/456 g)

- Blueberries (.25 cup/25 g)

- Liquid stevia (10 drops)

- MCT oil (2 tbsp.)

- Xanthan gum (.25 tsp.)

- Banana extract (1.5 tsp.)

- Ice cubes (2-3)

**Preparation Technique:**

1.  Measure and toss all of the fixings into a blender.

2.  Wait a few minutes for the seeds and flax to absorb some of the liquid.

3.  Pulse for one to two minutes until well combined and the texture you choose.

4.  Lastly, add the ice as desired before serving.

# Blueberry Essence

**Servings**: 1

**Nutritional Facts Per Serving**:

- Protein Counts: 31 g

- Total Fats: 21g

- Calories: 343

- Net Carbohydrates: 3 g

**Ingredients**:

- Coconut milk (1 cup/240 g)

- Blueberries (.25 cup/25 g)

- Vanilla Essence (1 tsp.)

- MCT oil (1 tsp.)

- Ice cubes (2-3)

**Preparation Technique:**

1. For a quick burst of energy, combine each of the fixings in a blender.

2. Puree until it reaches the desired consistency.

3. Pour and serve into a chilled glass.

# Cinnamon Smoothie

**Servings**: 1

**Nutritional Facts Per Serving**:

- Protein Counts: 24 g

- Total Fats: 40 g

- Calories: 467

- Net Carbohydrates: 5 g

**Ingredients**:

- Cinnamon (.5 tsp.)

- Coconut milk (.5 cup/114 g)

- Water (.5 cup/118 g)

- Extra-Virgin coconut oil/MCT oil (1 tbsp.)

- Ground chia seeds (1 tbsp.)

- Plain or vanilla whey protein (.25 cup/24 g)

- Optional: Stevia drops (to taste)

**Preparation Technique:**

1. Pour the milk, cinnamon, protein powder, and chia seeds in a blender.

2.  Empty the coconut oil, ice, and water.

3.  Add a few drops of stevia if desired.

# Smoothie in A Bowl

**Servings**: 1

**Nutritional Facts Per Serving**:

- Protein Counts: 35 g

- Total Fats: 35 g

- Calories: 570

- Net Carbohydrates: 4 g

**Ingredients**:

- Almond milk (.5 cup/120 g)

- Spinach (1 cup/30 g)

- Heavy cream (2 tbsp.)

- Low-carb protein powder (1 scoop)

- Coconut oil (1 tbsp.)

- Ice (2 cubes)

  *The Toppings:*

- Walnuts (4)

- Raspberries (4)

- Chia seeds (1 tsp.)

- Shredded coconut (1 tbsp.)

## Preparation Technique:

1. Add a cup of spinach to your high-speed blender. Pour in the cream, almond milk, ice, and coconut oil.

2. Blend for a few seconds until it has an even consistency, and all ingredients are well combined. Empty the goodies into a serving dish.

3. Arrange the toppings or give them a toss and mix them together. Of course, make it pretty and alternate the strips of toppings.

# Strawberry Avocado with Almond Milk

**Servings**: 5 - 1 cup each

**Nutritional Facts Per Serving**:

- Protein Counts: 1 g

- Total Fats: 8 g

- Calories: 106

- Net Carbohydrates: 7 g

**Ingredients**:

- Frozen strawberries (1 lb./455 g)

- Regular/vanilla Almond Breeze Original (.5 cup/120 g)

- Avocado (1 large)

- Powdered sweetener of choice (.25 cup/32 g or to taste)

**Preparation Technique:**

1. Prepare the smoothies in a blender until creamy and adjust the sweetener of choice to your liking.

Now, let us move on to how this all blends into a plan for one week!

# Chapter 9: 7-Day Meal Plan

Here is your balanced seven-day meal plan, which contains the total net carbs for each of the meal's components. Each one is based on the keto standards of 20-50 carbs daily. You can add additional snacks or desserts to your liking as long as you remain within your desired carb counts. Don't worry; if you do not see what you want, there are plenty of other recipes to choose from in the list of meals and snacks.

## Day 1:

**Breakfast: Healthy Bacon Hash & Eggs -** 9 g p.31

**Lunch: Tuna Salad & Chives -** 1 g p.39

**Dinner: Asparagus - Stuffed Chicken -** 2 g p.60

**Snack or Dessert: Raspberry Fudge -** 4.4 g p.105

## Day 2:

**Breakfast: Bagels & Cheese -** 8 g p.18

**Lunch: Steak Salad -** 1.5 g p.48

**Dinner: Spinach-Mozzarella Stuffed Burgers -** 1 g p.85

**Snack or Dessert: Chocolate Mousse -** 4 g p.98

## Day 3:

**Breakfast: Banana Pancakes -** 6.8 g p.19

**Lunch: Egg Drop Soup -** 3 g p.56

**Dinner: Jamaican Jerk Pork Roast -** 0 g p.88

**Snack or Dessert: Pumpkin Cheesecake with Almond Pecan Crust -** 6 g p.103

## Day 4:

**Breakfast: Coffee Cake -** 4 g p.29

**Lunch: Tuna Stuffed Avocado -** 3 g p.40

**Dinner: Green Beans & Chicken -** 4 g p.66

**Snack or Dessert: Chocolate Mini Cakes - Instant Pot -** 9 g p.97

## Day 5:

**Breakfast: Bacon & Avocado Omelet -** 3.3 g p.14

**Lunch: Keto Salad Niçoise -** 8 g p.46

**Dinner: Meatloaf -** 3 g p.81

**Snack or Dessert: Blueberry Cupcakes -** 2.8 g p.96

## Day 6:

**Breakfast: Choco-Breakfast Waffles -** 3.4 g p.27

**Lunch: No-Beans Chili Delight -** 5 g p.59

**Dinner: Basil Stuffed Chicken Breasts -** 1 g p.61

**Snack or Dessert: Pumpkin Bread -** 5 g p.102

# Day 7:

**Breakfast: Cream Cheese Eggs -** 3 g p.30

**Lunch: Avocado - Corn Salad -** 4.5 g p.41

**Dinner: Cabbage Skillet Tacos -** 4 g p.76

**Snack or Dessert: Almond Coconut Bars -** 2 g p.93

Now you truly see how easily you can remain on the ketogenic way of eating and not only remain unhungry; you will remain in ketosis and drop a few extra pounds with continued efforts.

You will need to formulate a game plan as you begin your ketogenic diet plan. That will include keeping track of your macronutrients. You can use any form you choose whether it is keeping a written journal or using an app. These are a few tips to get you started:

*Check Units of Measurement:* Many of the recipes you will discover over the Internet, or other sources may be listed in Imperial (ex. pounds) or in the Metric system.

*Standard Keto Calculator:* You will achieve the perfect mixture of the traditional keto diet plan of 5% carbs, 25% protein, and 70% ratios. (This is a general ratio.) Begin your weight loss process by making a habit of checking your levels when you want to know what essentials your body needs during the course of your dieting plan. You will document your personal information such as height and weight. The Internet calculator will provide you with essential math.

Be sure to remain diligent using the recipes as shown in each meal selection since it's practically impossible to precisely estimate the number of net carbs, fat, and protein in any given meal. Just be sure you've got the essential measuring tools on hand. This includes a kitchen scale, a good set of measuring spoons, and measuring cups.

Use glass containers for storing your prepared foods. Glass containers keep your food fresher longer. Plastic is cheaper, but the seal isn't as tight. Plastic can also cause your food to taste funky. Glass is overall a safer bet and worth the extra cost because plastic isn't always safe to use for reheating foods. If you use plastic, be sure it is a high-quality and trusted product that is safe for food storage and reheating.

Label the containers to make meal planning a breeze. There are some other things you have to consider when freezing your meals. You should always label your container with the date that you put it in the freezer. You also need to double check that your bottles, jars, or bags are each sealed tightly. If your containers aren't air-tight, your food will become freezer burnt and need to be trashed.

Freeze your meals so they will be ready when you are. For meals that are scheduled to be eaten at least three days after cooking, freezing is a great option. Freezing food is safe and convenient, but it doesn't work for every type of meal. You can also freeze the ingredients for a slow cooker meal and then just dump out the container into the slow cooker and leave it there. This saves a lot of time and means you can pre-prep meals up to one to two months in advance.

It can take up to two to three weeks or as much as a month before you achieve ketosis. After you've established that you're in ketosis, be sure to stick with your chosen method. If you cheat and go out of ketosis, it could take another month before your body is able to efficiently burn fat again. Cycling "in and out" of nutritional ketosis will maximize the natural benefits of cellular regeneration and renewal.

# Conclusion

I hope you have enjoyed each segment of *the Keto Diet*, let's hope it was informative and provided you with all of the tools you need to achieve your goals whatever they may be.

If you are focused on weight loss, the 7-Day meal plan will send you in the right direction. Making a few adjustments to your current kitchen stock can make the path much easier to keep those carbs at bay. Along with the guide, consider these substitutions to further your chances of success:

- *Flour:* Almond flour contains 3 grams of carbs for 1/4 of a cup. Coconut flour has 6 grams, but totals are overwhelming for the regular wheat flour at 24 grams. This is why it is not on your diet plan!

- *Breadcrumbs:* You can still enjoy your crunchiness by replacing regular breadcrumbs with crushed pork rinds. The good news is that the pork rinds have zero carbs. Next time enjoy healthier fats.

- *Pasta:* Replace pasta using zucchini. Use a spiralizer and make long ribbons to cover your plate. It is excellent for many dishes served this way.

- *Tortillas:* Get ready to say no to this one, which weighs in at approximately 98 grams for just one serving. Instead, enjoy a lettuce leaf at about one gram per serving. You will still have the 'healthy' crunch!

- *Regular Rice:* Replace the standard serving portions of white or brown rice with a portion of cauliflower rice.

You can exchange the 45 grams of carbs versus the 2.5 grams packed in for one cup of cauliflower rice.

- *Mashed Potatoes:* There's no need to prepare bowls of regular mashed potatoes. Instead, enjoy some mashed cauliflower.

## Enjoy These Snacks & Stay In Ketosis

Be sure to always have plenty of high-quality snacks waiting for those times when your resistance is down. When you choose snack items, always be sure to select ones that are low in carbs so your ketone levels will not be disrupted. If you have a busy lifestyle, pick some of the ones in the following list, but always remember to count the carbs.

- *Iced Coffee:* Leave the sugar out of your coffee and use only full-fat milk or cream. Add a bit of MCT oil powder, which can be purchased as chocolate, vanilla, or unflavored.

- *Beef Jerky:* Watch out for the added sugars. Choose ones with only a few additional ingredients.

- *Pork Rinds:* Use these to replace chips and crackers. For example, try Pork Clouds, which is a higher quality without a lot of offensive oil content.

- *Pepperoni Slices:* Enjoy the slices with a slice of high-fat cheese, but keep in mind, these are highly processed. Limit the amounts used and search for hormone-free or organic if possible.

- *Seaweed Snacks*: Search the labels to make sure they

do not contain significant amounts of oil.

- *String Cheese*: Choose the full-fat version without additional fillers.

- *Laughing Cow Cheese Wheels:* Purchase full-fat versions and get *real* cheese when possible.

- *Cacao Nibs*: You can enjoy the same crunch when used as an alternative to chocolate chips.

- *Stevia Sweetened Dark Chocolate*: If you are not using stevia, be sure it's a minimum of 80% or higher in cocoa content.

- *Sugar-Free Jell-O or Popsicles:* You can purchase this ready-to-go or make your own.

## Be Responsible Dining Out

Plan ahead before it's time to go out for dinner. Do some research before you leave the house. Many of the restaurants now have an online presence to make dieting while under ketosis much simpler. As you continue with your preplanning, it will become more natural, and you can branch out to other locations with the knowledge gained.

### Indian Cuisine

Indian cuisine is another delicious option for low-carb eaters. Ask for ghee/ clarified butter, which is an Indian staple made from pure fat. You can add it to any dish. You can also enjoy Indian homemade cheese but remember to watch out for hidden carbs. Thickeners and flour fixings are notorious for hidden carbs. Ask your waiter/waitress about the preparation methods.

Choose curries without potatoes, kebabs, and tandoori dishes. Maybe try some meat in creamy sauces such as tikka masala and butter chicken for a change. Avoid the portions, including the naan and rice. Instead, request some Raita, which is a creamy dip made from plain yogurt. It can be full-fat and served with some shredded cucumbers.

## Asian Cuisine

You will need to be careful when dining at Chinese, Japanese, Vietnamese, and Thai restaurants. Stay focused and don't order any items that taste sweet or ones that are battered. Ask your waiter to be sure, but you should be able to order a dish made with brown sauce. Curries and stir-fries that are made with low-carb vegetables, seafood, and meat are all excellent choices (no rice).

Request butter or coconut oil, which will add more fat to your diet. Peanut, olive oil, or sesame are another excellent option. Ask the waiter/waitress for the available options.

Enjoy your dinner meal with some crispy Duck. Be sure you do not use the sweet sauce. The same non-sweet logic applies to Chop Suey with no thickeners in the sauce, when possible. Shirataki noodles are a great low-carbohydrate choice if it's on the menu.

## How To Handle The Cravings

Do you know how to handle the cravings you will experience on the keto plan? These are a few to help keep your ketosis in line:

*Salty Foods:* If your body is craving foods such as pizza and chips, your body may be craving silicon. Have a few nuts and seeds; just be sure to count them into your daily counts. You may also be craving chloride or tryptophan. Munch on unsalted cottage cheese, cheese, fish, or spinach and add salt.

*Sugary Foods:* Several things can trigger the desire for sugar, but typically phosphorous, and tryptophan are the culprits. Have some chicken, beef, lamb, liver, cheese, cauliflower, or broccoli.

*Chocolate:* The carbon, magnesium, and chromium levels are requesting a portion of spinach, nuts, and seeds, or some broccoli and cheese. However, if you're craving chocolate, eat chocolate. You need to make sure you eat 75% or higher dark chocolate - not milk chocolate.

Finally, if you found this book useful in any way, a review on Amazon is always appreciated!

# Recipes Index


Asiago Bagels     25

Bacon & Avocado Omelet     27

Bacon - Egg & Cheese Cups     29

Bacon & Cheese Frittata     31

Bacon & Egg Muffins     33

Bagels & Cheese     35

Banana Pancakes     37

Biscuits & Gravy     39

BLT Wrap     41

Blueberry Scones     42

Breakfast Burrito     44

Brunch Zucchini Bread - Slow-Cooked     45

Butter Coffee     47

Cheesy Mushroom Omelet     48

Choco-Breakfast Waffles     50

Coconut-Almond Egg Wraps     52

Coffee Cake     54

Cream Cheese Eggs     56

Healthy Bacon Hash & Eggs — 57

Italian Cheesy Omelet — 59

Mackerel & Eggs — 61

1-Minute Keto Muffins — 63

Sesame - Poppy Seed Bagels — 65

Avocado - Tuna Melt Bites — 67

Baked Zucchini Noodles with Feta — 69

Ham & Spinach Mini Quiche — 71

Tuna Salad & Chives — 73

Tuna Stuffed Avocado — 74

Avocado - Corn Salad — 75

Caprese Salad — 77

Cobb Salad — 79

Deviled Chicken Salad Eggs — 81

Kale Parmesan Salad — 83

Keto Salad Niçoise — 84

Lobster Salad — 86

Steak Salad — 87

Thai Pork Salad — 89

Vegetarian Club Salad — 91

Asiago Tomato Soup ... 93

Beef & Carrot Soup - Instant Pot ... 95

Beef Stew ... 97

Chicken Chowder - Crockpot ... 99

Creamy Asparagus Soup ... 101

Egg Drop Soup ... 103

Kale - Sausage & Mushroom Soup ... 105

Mexican Chicken Soup - Slow-Cooked ... 107

No-Beans Chili Delight ... 109

Asparagus - Stuffed Chicken ... 111

Basil Stuffed Chicken Breasts ... 113

Cheesy Chicken Nuggets ... 115

Chicken Mozzarella & Pesto Casserole ... 117

Crack Chicken - Slow-Cooked ... 119

Creamy Onion Chicken ... 121

Preparation Technique: ... 121

Green Beans & Chicken ... 123

Kung Pao Chicken ... 125

Lemon Chicken with Angel Hair Pasta ... 127

Oven-Baked Pan-Fried Chicken ... 129

| | |
|---|---|
| Pizza Chicken Casserole | 131 |
| Rosemary Ranch Chicken Kabobs | 133 |
| Stuffed Chicken with Bacon & Asparagus | 135 |
| Bacon Burger Cabbage Stir Fry | 137 |
| Barbacoa Beef – Instant Pot | 139 |
| Beef Pizza | 141 |
| Cabbage Skillet Tacos | 143 |
| Cheesy Steak Pinwheels | 145 |
| Enchilada Skillet Dinner | 146 |
| Feta-Stuffed Burgers | 148 |
| Ground Beef Keto Meatballs | 150 |
| Meatloaf | 151 |
| Monterey Mug Melt | 153 |
| Skillet Steak - Nacho Style | 154 |
| Slow-Cooked London Broil | 156 |
| Spinach-Mozzarella Stuffed Burgers | 158 |
| Stroganoff | 160 |
| Bacon & Brussels Sprouts | 162 |
| Jamaican Jerk Pork Roast | 164 |
| Kalua Pork & Cabbage | 166 |

Pork Kabobs                                             168

Stuffed Pork Chops                                      170

Quick & Easy Lamb Chops                                 172

Almond Coconut Bars - Instant Pot                       174

Almond Pumpkin Seed Bars                                176

Amaretti Cookies                                        178

Blueberry Cupcakes                                      180

Chocolate Mini Cakes - Instant Pot                      182

Chocolate Mousse                                        184

Easy Brownie Inug                                       186

No-Bake Coconut Cashew Protein Bars                     187

Peanut Butter Protein Bars                              189

Pumpkin Bread                                           191

Pumpkin Cheesecake with Almond Pecan Crust              193

Raspberry Coke – Slow Cooker                            195

Raspberry Fudge                                         197

Strawberry & Cream Cakes                                199

Smoothies                                               201

Almond Lover Smoothie                                   201

Blueberry - Banana Bread Smoothie                       203

Blueberry Essence                                                    205

Cinnamon Smoothie                                                    206

Smoothie in A Bowl                                                   208

Strawberry Avocado with Almond Milk                                  210

# Description

Are you ready to take the plunge and begin your new way of living and eating?

Are you tired of trying fad diets that claim to work, but don't?

If so, you have made a huge step toward improving your lifestyle using the Ketogenic Diet Plan.

*Inside You Will Find:*

100 recipes to get you on the right path, including breakfast, lunch, dinner time, and snack-time recipes. You can choose between beef, poultry, pork, and so much more. If you are not convinced yet, these are just a few of the treats you will miss:

- Banana Pancakes

- Coffee Cake

- Asparagus - Stuffed Chicken

- Cobb Salad

- Feta-Stuffed Burgers Crack Chicken - Slow-Cooked

- Deviled Chicken Salad Eggs

- Vegetarian Club Salad

*What about some delicious desserts?*

- Pumpkin Cheesecake with Almond Pecan Crust

- Almond Pumpkin Seed Bars

- Raspberry Fudge

- Chocolate Mousse

*Does any of that sound like a diet? See for yourself!*

## Consider This: Who Can & Cannot Use the Ketogenic Techniques?

*Always, Check Your Medications for Compatibility:*

It's essential to inform your doctor about your weight loss program. He/she may prescribe some medicines that make you gain weight.

If you are taking insulin injections in high doses, your insulin can impede weight loss. By consuming fewer carbs, you are substantially reducing the requirement of insulin. Again, ask your healthcare professional before you make any changes.

*If You Are Attempting to Lose Weight: Be Aware Of Other Probable Medications Causing Weight Gain:*

- Oral contraceptives

- Antidepressants

- Epilepsy drugs

- Blood pressure medications

- Allergy medicines

- Antibiotics

If you enjoy working out for your health, be sure to do that at least four hours before sleeping. Make sure your room has sufficient darkness. You will wake refreshed, ready to face your tasty ketogenic breakfast.

*Do you take high blood pressure medications?* It's not your best move to begin a low-carb diet, including one like keto if you're currently taking other types of blood-pressure medications. If you feel weak, tired, or dizzy, you should check your blood pressure. If it's below 120/80, you should contact your physician to discuss a plan that's workable for you.

*Do you breastfeed?* You shouldn't participate in a low-carbohydrate diet plan, such as the ketogenic method. It's recommended to consume a minimum of 50 grams of carbs daily while breastfeeding. You can choose any way you like to get the extra carbs by selecting moderate and liberal low-carb recipes. Enjoy three fruits daily to boost your diet.

The high-fat and low-carb combination is a hit in this fabulous collection of desserts. The low-carbohydrate diet plan has many benefits, including:

- Its initial use of epilepsy

- Increased vitality and energy

- Accelerated fat loss

- Lowered blood sugar

- Lowered cholesterol

- Improved mental clarity or focus

Stay determined and stand by your goals during your transition to ketosis. Follow the instructions and recipe methods. Before long, you will be able to quickly scan other recipes and know before you finish reading how healthy they are for you and your family. The most significant benefit is that you are never hungry using the keto diet plan.

- *LeBron James:* This baller slimmed down and showed off his 6-pack in 2014 which he later revealed that the keto diet was the major influence of his success story. He didn't consume carbohydrates, sugar, or dairy products. It works!

- *Kim Kardashian:* Kim dropped over 50 pounds of baby weight on a Y low carb, ketogenic style diet by consuming less than 60 grams of carbs per day.

There is no need to wait. Why not get started on the path to a healthier outlook on life today! You know how to add this to your digital library. Let's Get Started!